7 STEPS TO ORGANIZATIONAL EXCELLENCE

A Practical, Interprofessional Approach to Evaluating Operations and Outcomes

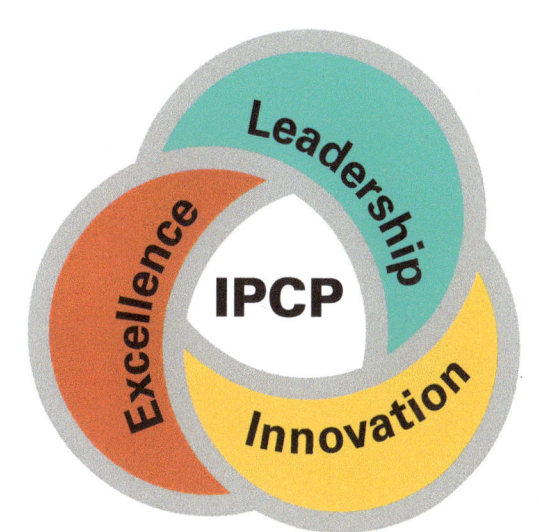

Nancy J. Robert, PhD, MBA, BSN

Managing Partner, Polaris Solutions

Kathy Chappell, PhD, RN, FNAP, FAAN

Senior Vice President of Accreditation, Certification, Measurement, & the Institute for Credentialing Research and Quality Management, American Nurses Credentialing Center

Susan D. Finlayson, DNP, RN, NE-BC

Senior Vice President of Operations, Mercy Medical Center

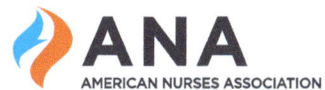

AMERICAN NURSES ASSOCIATION

American Nurses Association
8515 Georgia Avenue, Suite 400
Silver Spring, MD 20910-3492
1-800-274-4ANA

www.Nursingworld.org

Published October 2019

Print 978-1-947800-43-4
ePub 978-1-947800-44-1
EPDF 978-1-947800-45-8
Mobi 978-1-947800-46-5

TABLE OF CONTENTS

INTRODUCTION

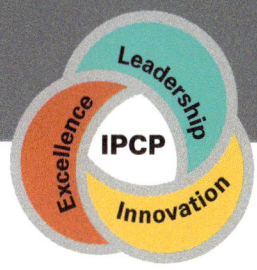

7 STEPS TO ORGANIZATIONAL EXCELLENCE

Health care today is experiencing fast, intense change and transformation. Everyone is grappling with an increasingly complex environment that requires innovative solutions to emerging health care opportunities. We all face heightened quality and safety imperatives, and we're continually challenged to attain higher levels of service and satisfaction. As expectations rise, we must find new ways to meet them.

The Institute of Medicine (IOM) report, *The Future of Nursing: Leading Change, Advancing Health*, emphasized the impact interprofessional collaboration has on improving accessibility, quality and the value of health care. With 29 million nurses and midwives participating in the delivery of global health care today, it is essential that organizations striving to achieve excellent patient and health system outcomes recognize that interprofessional collaboration and nursing excellence practices are indispensable to achieving the best possible healthcare outcomes.

Instilling nursing excellence practices as a component of interprofessional collaborative practice (IPCP) is the key to move forward with confidence. Organizations that develop and sustain a culture of nursing excellence embedded within collaborative team practices are in a prime position to advance fundamental principles that meet current health care delivery challenges while testing new principles that can drive the future of innovative health care delivery solutions.

Excellence starts with leadership and accelerates with innovations. But how do you successfully cultivate these core concepts to deliver exceptional performance and results? How do you ensure that organizational excellence practices are integrated into interprofessional team processes? How do you help your teams successfully deploy artificial intelligence and big data technologies that are changing health care?

This guide can help. It offers insights you need to achieve excellence every day. The guide is a companion piece to our *7 Steps to Organizational Excellence: A Practical,*

Interprofessional Approach to Evaluating Operations and Outcomes course, which provides IPCP, interprofessional education (IPE), and nursing healthcare leaders, healthcare consultants, and industry professionals with the knowledge and skills to help guide organizations to excellence. It provides an overview of excellence principles embedded in recognition programs such as ANCC's Magnet Recognition® and Pathway to Excellence®, and Accreditation programs that support nursing education, transition into practice, and interprofessional collaborative practice pursuits.

ANCC's recognition programs include interprofessional collaboration standards of excellence. The Magnet Recognition Program® is the highest organizational credential for nursing excellence, and the leading source of successful nursing practices and strategies worldwide. The Pathway to Excellence® designation is earned by healthcare organizations that measures the essential elements of an ideal nursing practice environment. The award substantiates the professional satisfaction of nurses and identifies best places to work. ANCC's Joint Accreditation™ program is the first and only innovation in the world offering multiple accreditations in one review process. Joint Accreditation™ promotes interprofessional continuing education (IPCE) activities specifically designed to improve interprofessional collaborative practice (IPCP) in health care delivery.

WHY WAS THE REFERENCE GUIDE CREATED?

The 7 Steps to Organizational Excellence book is all about you and your success. It's the ultimate reference guide to help you build organizational excellence into interprofessional collaborative practice teams as you pursue recognition programs or simply strive to achieve organizational performance goals. Regardless of why you elect to pursue organizational excellence, this guide can provide tips and tools to help you achieve your goals.

The guide includes practical, highly applicable tools to get your team energized around the necessary elements of forming IPCP teams, leadership essentials, innovation pathways, and mastering AI and big data concepts that are impacting health care today. We've included worksheets, exercises, templates, examples, relevant literature, and other real-world resources to help you assess your opportunities, implement meaningful changes, and evaluate your progress. Because each organization is different, the guide is meant as a way to help you generate your own ideas on how best to undertake your organizational excellence and interprofessional collaborative practice journey—you shape your own plan for success.

The guide ties excellence to critical priorities such as the Affordable Care Act measure domains and changing reimbursement policies from the Centers for Medicare & Medicaid Services. As you strengthen your demonstration of organizational excellence and interprofessional collaboration, you enhance your ability to quantify nursing's critical role in creating value and offering solutions in today's volatile environment.

For those who attend the *7 Steps to Organizational Excellence: A Practical, Interprofessional Approach to Evaluating Operations and Outcomes* course, this guide delivers continued support. It reinforces knowledge and relates recognition and accreditation principles to the modern healthcare landscape. You can use the resources provided to implement what you learn and apply concepts to everyday scenarios.

The guide is also an excellent introduction to ANCC's Magnet and Pathway to Excellence® Recognition Programs, and Accreditation and Certification opportunities that will help your organization excel. The guide highlights their many benefits, and how it can help your organization reach new levels of excellence in care delivery; practice environments; and high-quality patient, workforce, and organizational outcomes.

WHO IS IT FOR?

The *7 Steps to Organizational Excellence* book is designed for individuals and organizations seeking guidance on how to pursue organizational excellence and recommendations on how to embed those practices into interprofessional collaborative practice teams.

Whether you consult on healthcare issues, lead a healthcare organization, or simply want to learn more effective ways to advance quality and patient outcomes, the guide can help you understand the key variables that interact to create a culture of excellence and how to successfully embed those practices into interprofessional collaborative practice teams. It offers guidance to chief nursing officers, IPE and IPCP teams, Magnet, Pathway and Accreditation program directors, nurse leaders, and others who oversee patient care teams. It provides practical advice to healthcare consultants and industry executives who wish to connect with organizations seeking excellence outcomes, healthcare organizations interested in pursuing recognition programs such as Magnet and Pathway to Excellence, those seeking accreditation status for Joint CNE or Transition into Practice programs, or those organizations just interested in learning about organizational excellence concepts. And it serves as an easy-to-use roadmap to help healthcare organizations navigate the rapidly changing healthcare environment.

WHAT'S IN THE REFERENCE GUIDE?

STEP 1: Defining Excellence and Quality Outcomes

What is organizational excellence and how can it help you drive quality and outcomes? We share global health care perspectives from the United Nations 2030 Agenda for Sustainable Development Goal 3, *Good Health and Well-Being*, providing context about health care excellence and the impact on people's lives, take an in-depth look at the core elements of the U.S. National Quality Strategy health care priorities, present latest results from the Centers for Medicare & Medicaid Services (CMS) quality measure reporting system, explain how you can transform your environment to become a high performing organization prepared to meet the needs of the future, and take an in-depth look at the core elements of nursing excellence and interprofessional practice leadership factors.

The section features an overview of ANCC's Magnet Recognition Program, Pathway to Excellence, and Accreditation programs, and how they compare with other quality programs. Learn how the pursuit of interprofessional and nursing excellence can help your organization thrive in today's demanding consumer and regulatory environment.

STEP 2: Interprofessional Collaborative Practice (IPCP) and Interprofessional Education (IPE)

According to the World Health Organization, interprofessional collaborative practice (IPCP) happens "When multiple health workers from different professional backgrounds work together with patients, families, carers, and communities to deliver the highest quality of care." Why pursue IPCP in your organization? Because research demonstrates that effective interprofessional teams provide safer and higher quality patient care.

This step provides an overview of IPCP including strategies that interprofessional teams can implement to achieve success. Credentials such as those awarded to organizations (Magnet, Pathway, Accreditation), programs (Accreditation), and individuals (Certification) provide a framework as well as a validation mechanism of successful IPCP implementation.

Models of IPCP and interprofessional education (IPE) are presented, supported with resources available to help organizations succeed in IPCP initiatives.

STEP 3: Leadership—Building a Framework for Success

The Magnet Model and sources of evidence provide a framework to achieve excellence in nursing practice. Review the key components, then use the tools to conduct a gap analysis to assess your organization's strengths and opportunities in excellence, leadership and innovation.

A step-by-step template will help you craft a strategic plan that reflects your shared organizational vision and how to integrate it into the Magnet Model components that include interprofessional practice. We've included material that explains the value of a nursing professional practice model (PPM) to assess your nursing teams and drive interprofessional organizational excellence. Learn the basics and use the tools and examples provided to create an innovative PPM that aligns with your mission, vision, values, and strategic objectives that include how to work in interprofessional teams. Step 7 provides team tools to help you assess and implement new team processes that help you form a team of leaders.

STEP 4: Recognizing Team Readiness

Is your team ready to pursue excellence goals achieved by high-performing organizations? This step presents Nielson and Burns Four Developmental Levels Model (reactive, responsive, proactive, and high-performing), and how you can apply each one to the Magnet Model to achieve a more high-performing work environment. We share case studies and exemplars to help you assess the appropriate developmental level of your nursing workforce. Discover focused strategies to move your team, your division, or your entire organization to new levels of excellence.

Tools and team leadership exemplars to sharpen your leadership skills are included in Step 7.

STEP 5: Designing Your Innovation Journey

Find inspiration and creativity to achieve measurable results! Learn the basic concepts of innovation, review examples of the latest innovation models, and understand how the innovation gold rush will impact your organization. Explore the Global Innovation Index (GII) that distinguishes how countries stack up and learn about the 80 factors that can impact innovation progress. Assess how your organization's innovation strategy can help you navigate global drivers of health care innovation and gain perspective on "how to shoot for the moon."

Consider the eight indicators of extraordinary teams and assess your team's readiness to pursue innovation. Discover ways to maximize your environmental scan and assimilate the results into excellence models such as the Magnet Model. Identify outcomes to track the impact of innovation on patient care and organizational excellence. We provide tools and templates so you can map your innovation priorities to your strategic plan.

STEP 6: AI and Big Data—Opportunity or Danger?

Today there is no doubt that health care is experiencing rapid transformations that are accelerated by technology advancements. Health care applications are a leading industry in the digital revolution, with health care data accounting for about a third of the world's data. Of significant impact are artificial intelligence (AI) and big data—these technologies are changing the health care landscape. Why are these technologies now front and center? Because significant improvements in internet deployment, hardware, software and data science have provided opportunities to innovate new products and services that can solve real-world problems. This step explores what AI and big data are and how these technologies are impacting health care decision-making.

The world of health care is on a rapid pace of transformation aimed to provide better care, healthy people in healthy communities, and affordable care to all. AI and big data offer the promise of better insights through different thinking.

STEP 7: Tools and Resources

These are the resources that can help you build and implement a culture of organizational excellence.

DEFINING EXCELLENCE AND QUALITY OUTCOMES

STEP
1

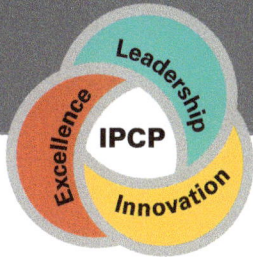

DEFINING EXCELLENCE AND QUALITY OUTCOMES

So, while the fundamental changes advocated by the Institute of Medicine (IOM) are unquestionably necessary, the systems changes that we bring about in our individual practices are both the place to begin and the level at which most of us can work. Large goals and principles are helpful as guides but, as in most things, change begins on the ground with each of us.

—Dr. John Frey III

INTRODUCTION OF EXCELLENCE CONCEPTS

This step explores organizational excellence and nursing's role in achieving excellence goals. How do we gauge excellence? An overview of the United Nations Member States' *2030 Agenda for Sustainable Development* goals provides context on global healthcare excellence and the impact on people's lives. As a United Nations member, the United States supports global healthcare goals and integrates some of the measures into national healthcare initiatives. Global health goals help shape our national healthcare agenda.

Our national healthcare agenda is managed by the Agency for Healthcare Research and Quality (AHRQ), which collaborates with agencies such as the Centers for Medicare & Medicaid Services (CMS) to identify, design, and implement relevant measures impacting healthcare progress. Each government agency has defined quality measures that are reported to Congress and to the public—the measures track our progress on achieving the nation's Triple Aim goals of better care, healthy people/healthy communities, and affordable care. In addition to CMS's priority measures that evaluate our nation's progress, reporting data from the Peterson-Kaiser Health System Tracker and the United Health Foundation's America's Health Rankings© annual report augments our understanding of our advancement toward achieving our nation's strategic healthcare priorities that now include measures for advancing care team well-being—healthcare's Quadruple Aim goals. The Health System

Tracker Dashboard provides trend information and insights about drivers and issues impacting healthcare delivery. The United Health Foundation annual report is in its 29th year of tracking 35 markers of community health status by state.

Recommendations regarding developing organizational excellence and high reliability models of care in healthcare settings are reviewed. An examination of nursing excellence concepts compared with ANCC's Magnet Recognition Program® model, Institute of Medicine (IOM) Core Competencies, Quality and Safety Education for Nurses (QSEN) Competencies, American Association of Critical-Care Nurses (AACH) Synergy Model for Patient Care®, and Institute for Healthcare Improvement (IHI) Always Event® models is discussed. The Magnet® Model is compared with Porter and Tanner's Organizational Excellence Framework to examine core themes of organizational excellence.

An overview of core principles embedded in the American Nurses Credentialing Center's global model for healthcare excellence is presented. Magnet and Pathway to Excellence® Recognition programs, and Accreditation programs that support interprofessional collaborative practice (IPCP) teams are offered as potential pathways to transform healthcare delivery and improve outcomes.

RECOMMENDED READING

Center for Clinical Standards and Quality, Centers for Medicare & Medicaid Services. (2018). *2018 National impact assessment of the Centers for Medicare & Medicaid Services (CMS) quality measures report.* Baltimore: Author. Retrieved from https://www.cms.gov/Medicare/Quality-Initiatives-Patient-Assessment-Instruments/QualityMeasures/Downloads/2018-Impact-Assessment-Report.pdf

Delivering quality health services: A global imperative for universal health coverage. (2018). Geneva: World Health Organization, Organization for Economic Co-operation and Development, and The World Bank. Retrieved from https://read.oecd-ilibrary.org/social-issues-migration-health/delivering-quality-health-services-a-global-imperative_9789264300309-en#page1

Ferguson, S. (2013). The global quest for nursing excellence. *Journal of Nursing Administration, 43*(11), 555–556.

IOM (Institute of Medicine). (2015). *Vital signs: Core metrics for health and health care progress.* Washington, DC: The National Academies Press.

HEALTHCARE EXCELLENCE DEFINED

In 2015 United Nations Member States adopted a *2030 Agenda for Sustainable Development,* a global initiative that defined a "shared blueprint for peace and prosperity for people and the planet, now and into the future. At its heart are the 17 Sustainable Development Goals (SDGs), which are an urgent call for action by all countries." The United Nations member states describe the goals as "the world's best plan to build a better world for people and our planet by 2030."[1]

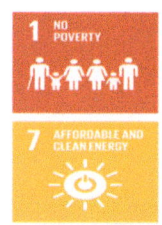 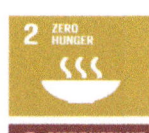 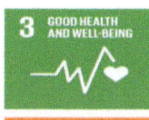  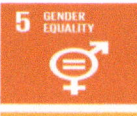 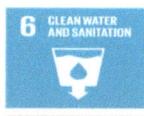 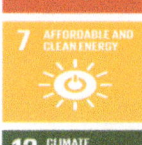 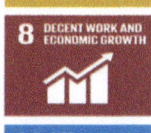 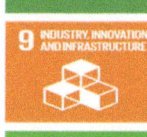 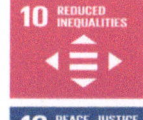 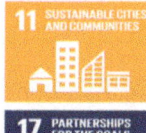    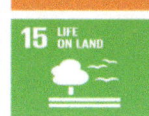 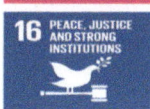 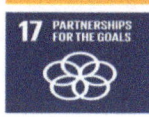 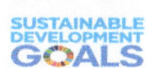

SDG 3: Good Health and Well-Being defines essential indicators that, if pursued, would provide outcomes that indicate targeted global population health and well-being standards of care delivery have been attained. SDG 3 targets maternal mortality; preventable deaths; ending epidemics such as AIDS, TB, and other communicable diseases; prevention and treatment to promote well-being while treating substance abuse; reducing deaths and injuries from road accidents; ensuring access to sexual and reproductive healthcare services; achieving universal health coverage to access safe, effective, quality, and affordable essential medicines and vaccines; and reducing deaths and illnesses from chemicals, air, water, and soil pollution. (See https://sustainabledevelopment.un.org/sdg3 for detailed health and well-being indicators.)

Health care and well-being are actively pursued through United Nations partnerships and country-specific health policies. A 2018 report, *Delivering Quality Health Services: A Global Imperative for Universal Health Coverage*, prepared by the World Bank, WHO, and OECD concluded that "optimal health care cannot be delivered by simply ensuring coexistence of infrastructure, medical supplies and health care providers. Improvement of health care delivery requires a deliberate focus on quality of health services, which involves providing effective, safe, people-centered care that is timely, equitable, integrated and efficient" (p. 11).[2]

Quality of care is the degree to which health services for individuals and populations increase the likelihood of desired health outcomes and are consistent with current professional knowledge.[2]

2018 GLOBAL ASSESSMENT OF QUALITY

Effectiveness—to evidence-based guidelines.

- Significant gap in provider knowledge and actual practice. Finding holds across all countries.

Patient Centered—needs/preferences are included in care.

- Differences between high-income and low-income countries in integrating this aspect into care.

Timeliness—waiting times vary by country and condition.

- Time to register for service and receive care significantly vary (example: hip replacement—42 days to 400 days).

Safety—unsafe practices are reduced.

- Cost of safety failures exceeds the cost of prevention.

Efficiency—resources are used appropriately.

- About 20%–40% of health resources are wasted.

Equity—delivery of care is equal across populations.

- Gaps exist everywhere with low-income populations more negatively impacted.

Integration—new dimension added in the 2018 report. Coordination for continuity of care is essential.

- Substantial gaps in all countries—coordination problems, lack of communication among providers.

EXHIBIT 1.1 CONTINUED

The IOM Model

In 2001, the Institute of Medicine put forth a framework that identified six core aims for a healthcare system to achieve quality outcomes.[3] In the United States today, this analytic framework drives the formulation of core measures of healthcare quality.[4]

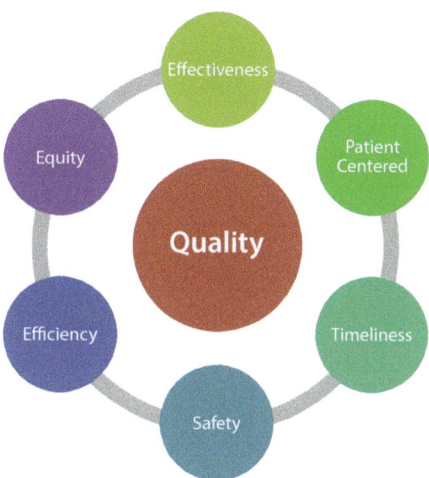

In the United States, the Agency for Healthcare Research and Quality (AHRQ) is a federal agency charged with improving the safety and quality of the US healthcare system. Its mission is to produce evidence to make health care safer, higher quality, more accessible, more equitable, and more affordable, and to team with other partners to make sure that the evidence is understood and used.[4]

With a 2019 budget of $451 million, it aims to provide education tools, innovation and measure support, and research on best practices.[5]

In the United States, healthcare excellence pursuits are defined by the 2001 IOM framework in Exhibit 1.1. The IOM framework now includes integrated care considerations. The 2018 SDG 3 global drivers of quality are highly aligned with the IOM framework.

Gaps were presented in the 2018 SDG 3 global assessment report on healthcare quality. The report identified four key actions listed in Table 1.1 that countries can pursue to improve progress on achieving healthcare quality.

TABLE 1.1
KEY ACTIONS FOR COUNTRIES TO IMPROVE QUALITY OUTCOMES

Develop, refine, and execute a national quality policy and strategy
Adopt and promote universal quality goals
Design a quality strategy that includes a set of quality interventions
Monitor and report quality of care results for continuous improvement efforts

Source: Delivering Quality Health Services: A Global Imperative for Universal Health Coverage (2018).

The 2018 SDG 3 Global Report concluded that, to be effective, implementation teams must include government agencies, health system leaders, patients, and clinicians that together design solutions that are supported by both patients and healthcare teams. Achieving healthcare excellence is a team endeavor—all participants must believe in and trust the healthcare system in order to make progress. To garner buy-in and trust, *transparency* about goals and measured outcomes is a critical first step to begin an excellence journey.

COMPONENTS OF HEALTHCARE EXCELLENCE

Achieving healthcare excellence requires clearly stated goals that are specific, timely, and measurable. Specific means that impacted constituencies have a role in determining what problems or issues are being addressed; timely in what expected actions will be required to achieve the goals within target dates; and measurable such that trend analysis can be used to gauge progress using a valid and reliable process.

In the United States, the pursuit of healthcare excellence is led by the Agency for Healthcare Research and Quality (AHRQ), an agency of the US Department of Health and Human Services (HHS). AHRQ has three primary objectives: (1) invest in quality research initiatives and disseminate evidence that improves quality, (2) create materials to train healthcare systems and providers on how to improve care, and (3) generate measures and data to track healthcare quality performance, and evaluate progress of the US healthcare system in achieving improvements in better health and better healthcare delivery. AHRQ leads National Quality Strategy (NQS) activities to identify meaningful measures and to evaluate progress.

In 2011, the NQS was the first national legislated effort to align public and private sector stakeholder goals to achieve better health and improved health care in America. The NQS collaborative process established three overarching aims supported by six common health priorities to guide healthcare quality efforts. The NQS was designed to be an evolving document—in 2016, nine "levers" were identified, each representing a core business function, resource, or action that stakeholders could use to achieve NQS goals. NQS aims, priorities, and levers are depicted in Exhibit 1.2. Stakeholders are identified in the outermost ring, with all contributing to achieving Healthy People, Better Care, and Affordable Care aims through the identification and definition of essential quality measures.

EXHIBIT 1.2

NATIONAL QUALITY STRATEGY AIMS, PRIORITIES, AND LEVERS

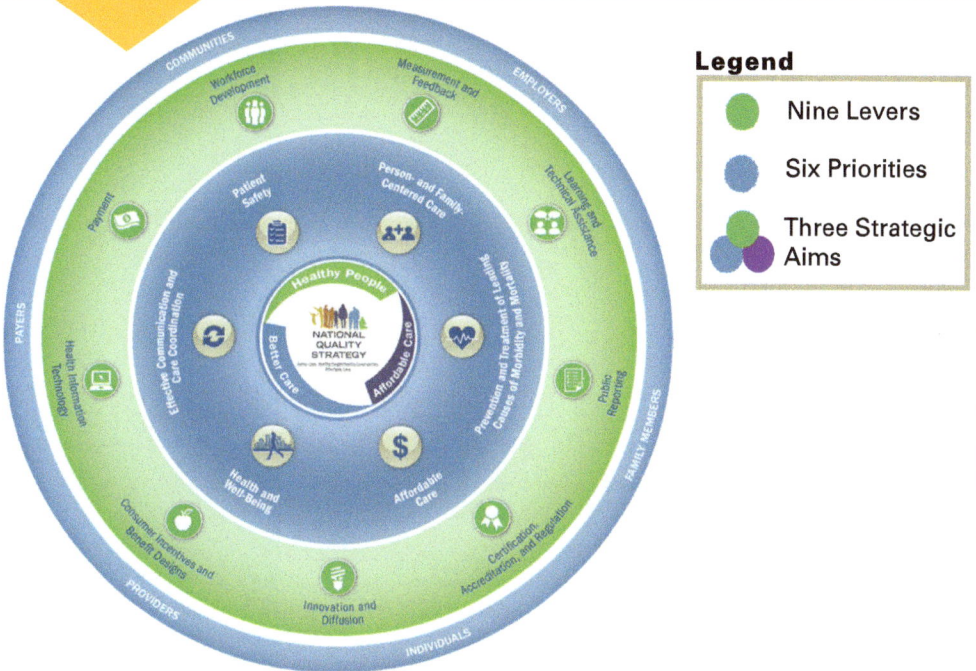

Legend

- Nine Levers
- Six Priorities
- Three Strategic Aims

Source: Slide Set: National Quality Strategy Overview. Content last reviewed January 2017. Agency for Healthcare Research and Quality, Rockville, MD. https://www.ahrq.gov/workingforquality/nqstools/briefing-slides.html

LEVER	LEVER DESCRIPTION
Measurement and Feedback	Provide performance feedback to plans and providers to improve care.
Learning/Technical Assistance	Foster learning environments that offer training, resources tools, and guidance to achieve quality goals.
Public Reporting	Compare treatment results, costs, and patient experience.
Certification, Accreditation, and Regulation	Adopt or adhere to approaches to meet safety and quality standards.
Innovation and Diffusion	Foster innovation in health care quality improvement, facilitate rapid adoption within and across organizations and communities.
Consumer Incentives, Benefit Designs	Help consumers adopt healthy behaviors and make informed decisions.
Health Information Technology	Improve communication, transparency, and efficiency for better coordinated health and health care.
Payment	Reward and incentivize provider to deliver high-quality, patient-centered care.
Workforce Development	Invest in people to prepare the next generation of health care professionals and support lifelong learning for providers.

Source: About the National Quality Strategy. Content last reviewed March 2017. Agency for Healthcare Research and Quality, Rockville, MD. https://www.ahrq.gov/workingforquality/about/index.html

NQS Priorities

The NQS focuses on six priorities that address the most common health concerns that Americans face. The priorities are:

 Making care safer by reducing harm caused in the delivery of care.

 Ensuring that each person and family is engaged as partners in their care.

 Promoting effective communication and coordination of care.

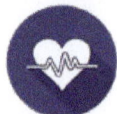 Promoting the most effective prevention and treatment practices for the leading causes of mortality, starting with cardiovascular disease.

 Working with communities to promote wide use of best practices to enable healthy living.

 Making quality care more affordable for individuals, families, employers, and governments by developing and spreading new health care delivery models.

Source: Agency for Healthcare Research and Quality. (2017). Introduction to the National Quality Strategy. OMB No. 17-0043-1-EF. Rockville, MD: Author. Retrieved from https://www.ahrq.gov/workingforquality/nqs-tools/alignment-toolkit.html

Who decides which healthcare measures are essential for achieving Triple Aim goals and priorities? How are measurement standards defined, deployed, tested, and revised?

Under the Patient Protection and Affordable Care Act (ACA), the Centers for Medicare & Medicaid Services (CMS) is one agency charged with driving quality improvements in national health care through priority goals as displayed in Exhibit 1.2. CMS collaborates with AHRQ and other stakeholders to define, develop, disseminate, and document progress on existing and new measures.

Who decides which healthcare organizations and practitioners meet national healthcare standards?

Federal agencies such as CMS drive compliance through federally mandated reimbursement practices. Insurance carriers are implementing novel ways to negotiate payments based on patient health outcomes that meet established measures. Most importantly, patients are impacting the delivery of services through their participation and input on healthcare provider assessment tools. Results are located on sites such as CMS Physician Compare (https://www.medicare.gov/physiciancompare/#search)—a public site mandated in 2010 in the Affordable Care Act—that provide information on physicians and physician groups that participate in quality measure programs and display results of Consumer Assessment of Healthcare Providers and Systems (CAHPS) surveys. CAHPS highlight patient experiences with physicians or physician groups, and each provider can earn merit-based incentives. (See https://www.cms.gov/research-statistics-data-and-systems/research/cahps/index.html for a detailed list of CMS-approved CAHPS survey instruments for various health providers that include physicians, nurse practitioners, physician assistants, and health systems.)

EXERCISE 1.1 — UNDERSTANDING MEASURES AND MEASURE SOURCES, PART 1

1. In 2018 the six national priorities tracked 533 implemented measures aimed toward identifying components of high-quality care. Access the detailed CMS Measure List Tool at https://cmit.cms.gov/CMIT_public/ListMeasures.

    a. Select **Programs** then select **Healthcare Priority** from the sidebar.

    b. From the **Filter** by Healthcare Priority page **Select** measure 'Ensure that each person and family are engaged as partners in their care (1)'.

    c. Select **Apply Filter**.

    d. Click on the underlined **Measure Title**. See a report generated about the measure.

2. When you are ready, **EXPORT** the PDF report from the online screen. Explore each tab (PROPERTIES, STEWARD, CHARACTERISTICS, GROUPS, PROGRAMS, LINKS, SIMILAR MEASURES).

    • Do you understand what the measure is and how it is measured?

    • Do the tabs provide measure transparency and is the data presented actionable?

    • Does the measure meet the 2018 Global Assessment on Health Care Quality Key Actions criteria for monitoring and reporting as listed in Table 1.1?

In 2017, a new CMS initiative, Meaningful Measures, was launched. The purpose of the program is to provide a new framework for CMS to identify priorities for quality measurement and improvement that are most critical to providing high-quality care and improving individual outcomes. The program was launched based on a recognized need to improve outcomes for patients, reduce the data reporting burden and costs on healthcare providers, and focus quality measurement efforts to better align with what is meaningful to patients. Following public input, a total of 19 Meaningful Measure Areas were identified and are detailed in Table 1.2.

According to the CMS Meaningful Measures Hub,

> Meaningful Measures is not intended to replace existing programs but will help programs identify and select individual measures. Meaningful Measure areas are intended to increase measure alignment across CMS programs and other public and private initiatives. Additionally, it will point to high priority areas where there may be gaps in available quality measures while helping guide CMS's effort to develop and implement quality measures to fill those gaps.

TABLE 1.2
2018 MEANINGFUL MEASURES

MEANINGFUL MEASURE AREA	NQS PRIORITIES	DESCRIPTION
Healthcare-Associated Infections	Making Care Safer by Reducing Harm Caused in the Delivery of Care	On any given day, about 1 in 25 hospital patients has at least one healthcare-associated infection. Prevent healthcare-associated infections that occur in all health-care settings.
Preventable Healthcare Harm	Making Care Safer by Reducing Harm Caused in the Delivery of Care	Each year, 2.8 million people are treated in emergency departments for fall injuries, with associated costs of $31 billion. Avoid non-infectious harms like falls and complications like bed sores; harm that occurs during care is a leading cause of significant morbidity and mortality and occurs in both inpatient and outpatient settings.
Care Is Personalized and Aligned with Patient's Goals	Strengthen Person and Family Engagement as Partners in Their Care	"Researchers have been using goal-attainment scaling for decades to measure the effect of treatment for conditions such as dementia and for comprehensive geriatric assessments." Ensure the care delivered is in concert with individual's goals, aligned with the care plan co-created with their doctor, and evidenced by people making informed decisions about their care.
End of Life Care According to Preferences	Strengthen Person and Family Engagement as Partners in Their Care	Fewer than 50% of even severely or terminally ill patients have an advance directive in their medical record. Ensure that care delivered at the end of life is in concert with patient/family preferences, which includes knowing those desires and providing aligned care and services.

MEANINGFUL MEASURE AREA	NQS PRIORITIES	DESCRIPTION
Patient's Experience of Care	Strengthen Person and Family Engagement as Partners in Their Care	Recent average positive reports of healthcare experiences showed variation across a range of factors, for example, from 52% for "Care transitions" to 87% for "Discharge information." Actively engage patients in reporting their experiences including satisfaction with care and staff, and community inclusion.
Patient Reported Functional Outcomes	Strengthen Person and Family Engagement as Partners in Their Care	Slightly more than 15% of adults report physical-functioning difficulties. Improve or maintain patient's quality of life by addressing physical functioning that affects their ability to undertake daily activities most important to them.
Medication Management	Promote Effective Communication and Coordination of Care	Annual healthcare costs in the United States from adverse drug events (ADEs) are estimated at $3.5 billion, resulting in 7,000 deaths annually. Avoid medication errors, drug interactions, and negative side effects by reconciling and tailoring prescriptions to meet the patient's care needs.
Admissions and Readmissions to Hospitals	Promote Effective Communication and Coordination of Care	Nearly 1 in 5 Medicare fee-for-service hospital discharges have previously resulted in a readmission within 30 days, accounting for more than $17 billion in avoidable Medicare expenditures. Prevent unplanned admissions and readmissions to the hospital; unplanned admissions and readmissions have negative impacts on patients, caregivers, and clinical resources, and can be prevented with effective care coordination and communication.
Transfer of Health Information and Interoperability	Promote Effective Communication and Coordination of Care	Fewer than 10% of physicians have fully functional electronic medical record/electronic health record (EMR/EHR) systems. Promote interoperability to ensure current and useful information follows the patient and is available across every setting and at each healthcare interaction.
Preventive Care	Promote Effective Prevention and Treatment of Chronic Disease	Many screening rates, like those for cancer, are below desired levels and reflect disparities across ethnicity/race. Prevent diseases by providing immunizations and evidence-based screenings, and promoting healthy lifestyle behaviors and addressing maternal and child health.
Management of Chronic Conditions	Promote Effective Prevention and Treatment of Chronic Disease	People with multiple chronic conditions account for 93% of total Medicare spending. Promote effective management of chronic conditions, particularly for those with multiple chronic conditions.
Prevention, Treatment, and Management of Mental Health	Promote Effective Prevention and Treatment of Chronic Disease	Annually, 1 in 5 or 43.8 million adults in the U.S. experience mental illness. Diagnosis, prevention, and treatment of depression and effective management of mental disorders (e.g., schizophrenia, bipolar disorder) and dementia (e.g., Alzheimer's disease) with emphasis on effective integration with primary care.
Prevention and Treatment of Opioid and Substance Use Disorders	Promote Effective Prevention and Treatment of Chronic Disease	Annually, 3 out of 5 drug overdose deaths involve an opioid, resulting in over $72 billion in medical costs. Ensure screening for and treatment of substance use disorders, including those co-occurring with mental health disorders.

MEANINGFUL MEASURE AREA	NQS PRIORITIES	DESCRIPTION
Risk-Adjusted Mortality	Promote Effective Prevention and Treatment of Chronic Disease	Heart disease, cancer, and chronic lower respiratory diseases are among the leading causes for death. Reduce mortality rate for patients in all healthcare settings.
Equity of Care	Work with Communities to Promote Best Practices of Healthy Living	In 2015, compared to 1996, children and adults were more likely to visit a health provider. Ensure high-quality and timely care with equal access for all patients and consumers, including those with social risk factors, for all health episodes in all settings of care.
Community Engagement	Work with Communities to Promote Best Practices of Healthy Living	It is estimated that a $10 per person per year investment in community-based programs could save $16 billion in medical cost savings per year reflective of improved health. Increase the use and quality of home- and community-based services (HCBS) to promote public health including a focus on health literacy.
Appropriate Use of Healthcare	Make Care Affordable	Overuse of services is estimated to account for nearly $300 billion a year in expenditures. Ensure patients receive the care they need while avoiding unnecessary tests and procedures.
Patient Focused Episode of Care	Make Care Affordable	Approximately 30% of healthcare spending is for services without health benefits to patients. Improve care by optimizing health outcomes and resource use associated with treating acute clinical conditions or procedures.
Risk-Adjusted Total Cost of Care	Make Care Affordable	In 2015, Medicaid spent $545.1 billion and Medicare spent $646.2 billion, with over 400 Medicare ACOs contributing more than $466 million in total program savings. Hold healthcare providers accountable for the total costs of care to mitigate out-of-pocket costs to the patient, lower costs to the Medicare program, ensure efficient use of high-value services, improve the quality of care, and safeguard the future of services and programs, with a focus on price transparency and continual improvements in quality.

Source: CMS Initiatives Meaningful Measures Hub, 2018.

The creation of a national quality agenda was driven by a need to improve healthcare delivery and patient outcomes.[6] The Institute of Medicine's 1999 seminal report ignited a call to action in the healthcare community, and the 2015 RAND Corporation assessment of our progress estimated that more than 580 health-related organizations disseminated quality measures that included many CMS measures.[7] If Meaningful Measures are successful, it is expected that we will have shifted our attention to measurement efforts that promulgate a patient-centered healthcare framework. (See Exercise 1.2.)

Previous measurement efforts set the stage for healthcare providers and patients to pilot new ways to deliver, measure, and assess healthcare outcomes. Our next challenge is to take what we have learned in healthcare delivery over the last two decades and pursue new approaches to deliver healthcare services that get in front of illness, shifting our focus to pursuits that keep us healthy. Changes in treatment options, provider abilities, patient

1. In 2017, nineteen Meaningful Measures were integrated into NQS indicators. Access the detailed CMS Measure List Tool at https://cmit.cms.gov/CMIT_public/ListMeasures.

   a. Select **Meaningful Measure Area**.

   b. From the **Filter** by Meaningful Measure Area page **Select** 'Care is Personalized and Aligned with Patient's Goals (19)' from the right sidebar. Click on **Apply Filter**.

   c. Scroll down the page and note the different measures associated with this goal. Move from left to right and examine each column header. Note the different programs a measure can support.

   d. Click on the **3-Item Care Transition Measure**. See a report generated about the measure.

2. When you are ready, **EXPORT** the PDF report from the online screen. Explore each tab (PROPERTIES, STEWARD, CHARACTERISTICS, GROUPS, PROGRAMS, LINKS, SIMILAR MEASURES, ENVIRONMENTAL SCAN).

   • Do you understand what the measure is and how it is measured?

   • Does the assigned Meaningful Measure category seem accurate? Useful?

   • Does your organization report on Meaningful Measures?

engagement, and technology are propelling delivery transformations in unique and unpredictable ways—this sets the stage for designing the next generation of healthcare options that deliver on Healthy People, Better Care, and Affordable Care.

The delivery of health care is complex, highly diversified, and professionally complicated. The goal is to deliver high-quality care at the right time, in the right venue, offering effective and integrated treatment support, while responding to a patient's needs and preferences and taking into account safe practices. The healthcare profession takes on this audacious goal in order to achieve the best possible health outcomes. We are clear about the direction we seek, but according to the CMS *2018 Quality Measures Report*,[8] the Peterson-Kaiser Health Tracker Dashboard,[9] and the United Health Foundation's *America's Health Rankings©* *2018 Annual Report*,[10] healthcare systems have made progress but continue to find it challenging to achieve targeted outcomes across healthcare offerings in a variety of community settings.

2018 CMS Impact Report Findings

Every three years under the Department of Health and Human Services, CMS assesses and reports to Congress the impact and use of endorsed quality measures that support a variety of healthcare programs across multiple agencies. The report is required under section 1890A(a)(6) of the Social Security Act.

Of the 762 unique measures available (see Exhibit 1.3), *The 2018 Impact Report*'s initial analysis included 253 measures that had three or more years of data available. The initial trend analysis represented 33% of total CMS measures currently tracked. Of the 253 measures tracked, 62 (25%) were included in the final 2018 impact report. Each measure was evaluated using 2015 baseline figures.

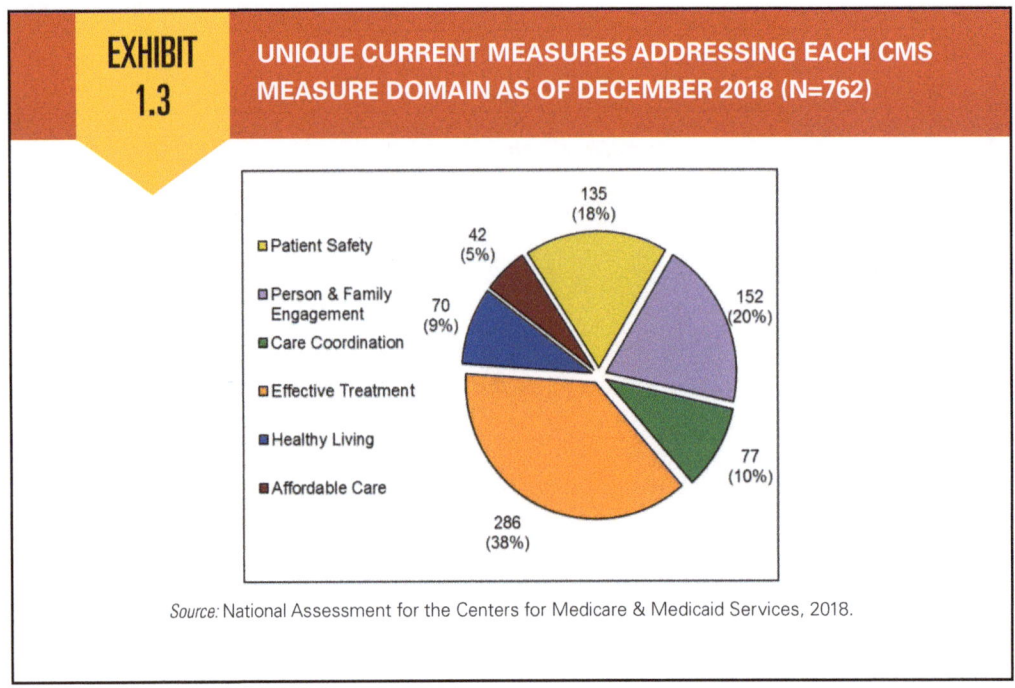

EXHIBIT 1.3

UNIQUE CURRENT MEASURES ADDRESSING EACH CMS MEASURE DOMAIN AS OF DECEMBER 2018 (N=762)

- Patient Safety
- Person & Family Engagement
- Care Coordination
- Effective Treatment
- Healthy Living
- Affordable Care

135 (18%)
42 (5%)
70 (9%)
152 (20%)
77 (10%)
286 (38%)

Source: National Assessment for the Centers for Medicare & Medicaid Services, 2018.

Measures were identified as +1% improvement (green), −1% declining (red), stable (orange), and ≥10% improving rapidly (as noted on dashboards). The 62 measures analyzed in the final 2018 report presented to Congress represent about 8% of total CMS measures in use today. (See Table 1.3.)

While the 2018 CMS report provides guideposts regarding our progress since 2012, healthcare delivery progress is also monitored by external groups such as the Peterson-Kaiser Health System Tracker, United Health Foundation's American's Health Rankings© annual report, and numerous healthcare advocacy groups including the National Quality Forum, OECD Stat Global Health Statistics, and patient advocacy groups such as the

TABLE 1.3

2018 NATIONAL HEALTH PRIORITY MEASURES REPORTED TO CONGRESS

NATIONAL HEALTH PRIORITY	GREEN (IMPROVING)	ORANGE (STABLE)	RED (DECLINING)	NUMBER OF CMS MEASURES EVALUATED IN 2018 REPORT/ (% OF ALL CMS MEASURES IN EACH PRIORITY CATEGORY*)
Patient Safety	6	2	3	11/(8%)
Person and Family Engagement	7	11	0	18/(12%)
Care Coordination	2	3	0	5/(7%)
Effective Treatment	7	3	1	11/(4%)
Healthy Living	14	1	1	16 (2 with insufficient data)/ (23%)
Affordable Care	0	0	1	1 – Increasing Costs/ (2%)

*Data figures rounded for each priority category

Total Current Measures for CMS Measure Domains as of December 2018 (n=762). Each National Health Priority domain varies in number of measures in use. See Exhibit 1.3 for details.

American Cancer Society, the National Patient Safety Foundation, and Institute for Health Improvement (IHI). These groups seek to engage healthcare teams, patients, and families in achieving high-quality healthcare outcomes by using evidence to shape health policy and regulatory statutes, and to engage consumers in establishing healthcare delivery expectations and consumer responsibilities in healthcare consumption.

To highlight how alternative data sources can provide insight about NQS progress, let's examine the CMS priority of Affordable Care. The 2018 CMS report noted that costs were increasing but did not provide further indices as to how this impacts consumer healthcare costs. The Peterson-Kaiser Health System Tracker Dashboard illuminates what is occurring across the nation regarding shifting healthcare costs to consumers.

Consumers are worried about healthcare expenditures that are unexpected, such as new co-pays and deductibles, and have experienced the impact of rising out-of-pocket (OOP) costs. In 2017, average OOP expenses for those with employer-based healthcare plans totaled $791. This represents an increase of 68% in expenses shifted to employees since 2006. Exhibit 1.4 displays the Peterson-Kaiser Rising Deductibles analysis that highlights key concerns impacting healthcare consumers. While co-pays are decreasing, deductibles and co-insurance amounts continue to rise.[11]

A provision of the 2010 Affordable Care Act mandated that each hospital operating within the United States shall for each year establish (and update) and make public (in accordance with guidelines developed by the HHS secretary) a list of the hospital's standard charges for items and services provided by the hospital.[12] In April 2018, the HHS secretary announced the requirement for a January 1, 2019, implementation of the ACA mandate, with the goal to provide consumers price transparency. Hospitals responded to the mandate by dumping

EXHIBIT 1.4 — OUT-OF-POCKET SPENDING ANALYSIS

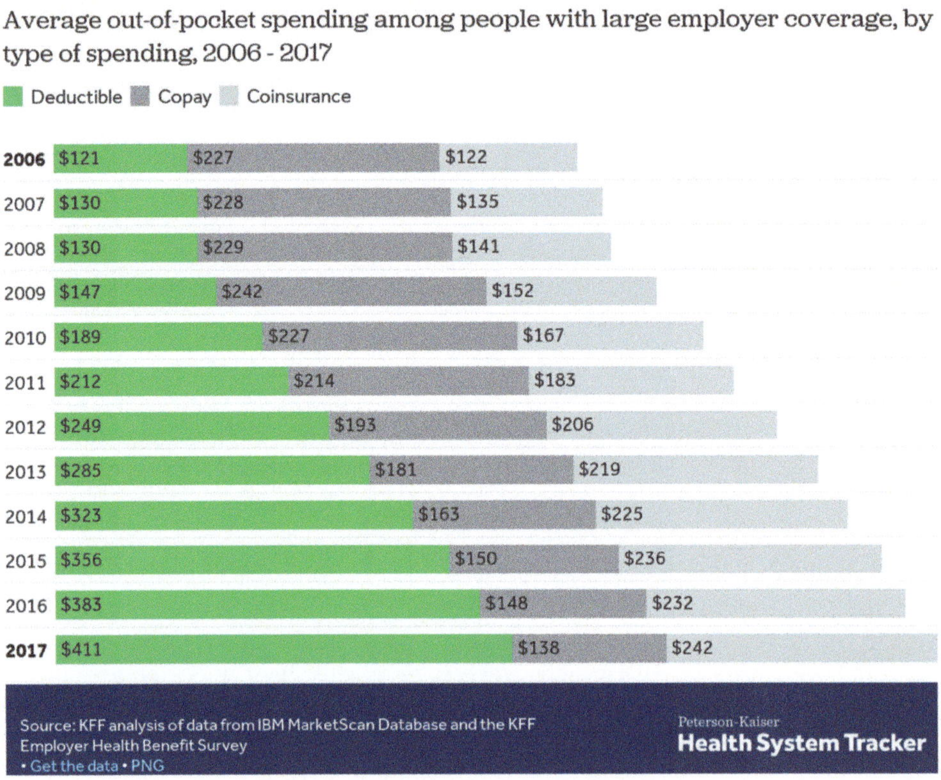

Average out-of-pocket spending among people with large employer coverage, by type of spending, 2006 - 2017

■ Deductible ■ Copay ■ Coinsurance

Year	Deductible	Copay	Coinsurance
2006	$121	$227	$122
2007	$130	$228	$135
2008	$130	$229	$141
2009	$147	$242	$152
2010	$189	$227	$167
2011	$212	$214	$183
2012	$249	$193	$206
2013	$285	$181	$219
2014	$323	$163	$225
2015	$356	$150	$236
2016	$383	$148	$232
2017	$411	$138	$242

Source: KFF analysis of data from IBM MarketScan Database and the KFF Employer Health Benefit Survey
• Get the data • PNG

Peterson-Kaiser Health System Tracker

Rae, M., Cox, C., Claxton, G., & Levitt, L., (Deductible relief day: How rising deductibles are affecting people with employer coverage, (Peterson-Kaiser Health System Tracker, [May 15, 2019]).

chargemaster lists with 10,000-plus line items described in undecipherable terms onto internet sites. Even if a consumer could find all the line items associated with a specific hospital service, the chargemaster charges may not be relevant to a specific consumer because healthcare plans dictate different terms of cost sharing and payments rendered to a hospital for each procedure or service. The consequence of the mandate was that consumers were deluged with meaningless information.

Another Peterson-Kaiser finding is that cost of care seems to be location dependent.[9] An analysis of expenditures by selected procedures highlights why it is difficult for consumers to understand prices for services rendered. For example, while the 2016 national average cost of employer insurance payments for a total knee replacement was $34,063, Exhibit 1.5 highlights variances in prices based on geographic location. To add further complexity, within a geographic location prices can also vary among healthcare delivery sites.

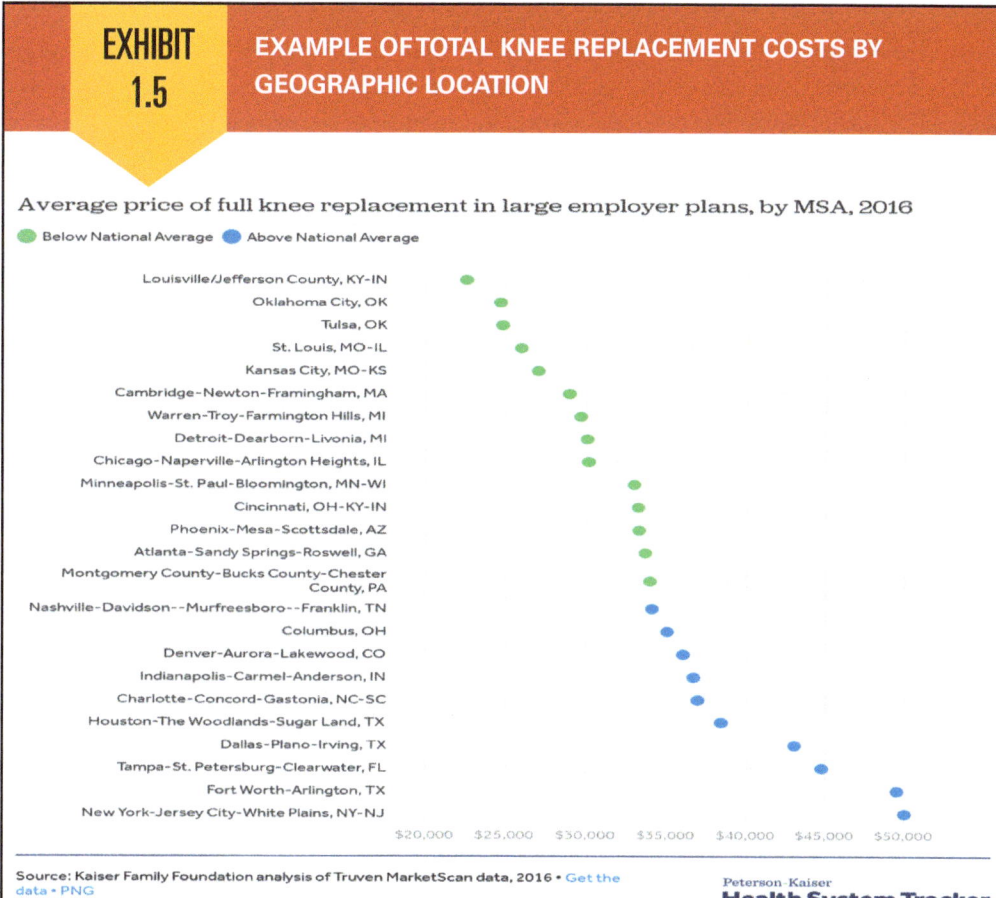

EXHIBIT 1.5

EXAMPLE OF TOTAL KNEE REPLACEMENT COSTS BY GEOGRAPHIC LOCATION

Average price of full knee replacement in large employer plans, by MSA, 2016

● Below National Average   ● Above National Average

Louisville/Jefferson County, KY-IN	
Oklahoma City, OK	
Tulsa, OK	
St. Louis, MO-IL	
Kansas City, MO-KS	
Cambridge-Newton-Framingham, MA	
Warren-Troy-Farmington Hills, MI	
Detroit-Dearborn-Livonia, MI	
Chicago-Naperville-Arlington Heights, IL	
Minneapolis-St. Paul-Bloomington, MN-WI	
Cincinnati, OH-KY-IN	
Phoenix-Mesa-Scottsdale, AZ	
Atlanta-Sandy Springs-Roswell, GA	
Montgomery County-Bucks County-Chester County, PA	
Nashville-Davidson--Murfreesboro--Franklin, TN	
Columbus, OH	
Denver-Aurora-Lakewood, CO	
Indianapolis-Carmel-Anderson, IN	
Charlotte-Concord-Gastonia, NC-SC	
Houston-The Woodlands-Sugar Land, TX	
Dallas-Plano-Irving, TX	
Tampa-St. Petersburg-Clearwater, FL	
Fort Worth-Arlington, TX	
New York-Jersey City-White Plains, NY-NJ	

$20,000 $25,000 $30,000 $35,000 $40,000 $45,000 $50,000

Source: Kaiser Family Foundation analysis of Truven MarketScan data, 2016 • Get the data • PNG

Peterson-Kaiser
Health System Tracker

Claxton, G., Rae, M., Levitt, L., Cox, C & Kaiser Family Foundation, How have healthcare prices grown in the U.S. over time?, (Peterson-Kaiser Health System Tracker, [May 8, 2018])

An example of comparative state-by-state data related to CMS Meaningful Measures priorities concerned with Promoting Effective Treatment can be found in United Health Foundation's America's Health Rankings© annual report.[10] A current CMS measure goal of Healthy Weight is measured by body mass index (BMI) screening and follow-up. The America's Health Rankings report identifies state obesity statistics by education level and pinpoints gaps requiring attention. The report delves further into conditions related to obesity, such as physical inactivity, that may be a contributing factor in mitigating obesity. The state-by-state measures allow states to better understand unique population needs that can drive actionable preventive measures.

Given the complexity of healthcare pricing, is it really reasonable to assume that consumers will be able to navigate healthcare cost structures on their own? Jeanne Pinder, CEO and founder of ClearHealthCosts.com, believes a system based on real world experience of prices charged will accelerate healthcare cost transparency. She created a website that crowdsources itemized cost experiences for common services rendered such as MRIs. Armed with real world data, she believes consumers will take actions necessary to control healthcare costs by purchasing from quality providers who offer reasonable prices. With healthcare costs taking a larger portion of wages, the healthcare industry has attracted consumer awareness and sensitivity about healthcare prices. The HHS secretary believes that transparent healthcare pricing will eventually drive down costs, and the Trump administration's April 2018 mandate was an effort to begin the process.

HEALTHCARE QUALITY MEASURES—DO THEY MAKE A DIFFERENCE?

An old adage by Peter Drucker, management expert, states "What gets measured gets managed." According to 2015 and 2018 evaluation of quality measures reports commissioned by CMS, it seems that Drucker's supposition is correct. The 2015 and 2018 *National Impact Assessment of the Centers for Medicare & Medicaid Services (CMS) Quality Measures Reports* conclude that implementing measures does make a difference in achieving healthcare quality outcomes, and that CMS quality measures positively affect Medicare, Medicaid, and the Children's Health Insurance Program (CHIP), as well as other payer sources.

ACHIEVING EXCELLENCE IN HIGH-PERFORMING ORGANIZATIONS

What differentiates a high-performing healthcare organization? How do organizations achieve and maintain standards of excellence over time and across a variety of competitive conditions? How do healthcare systems successfully navigate the complex healthcare environment to become a high-reliability organization?

> *According to the American Society for Quality, an organization founded in 1946 to promote quality principles worldwide,* **organizational excellence** *is defined as "the ongoing efforts to establish an internal framework of standards and processes intended to engage and motivate employees to deliver products and services that fulfill customer requirements within business expectations. It is the achievement by an organization of consistent superior performance—for example, outputs that exceed meeting objectives, needs, or expectations."[13]*

Organizational excellence principles provide foundational steps that support efforts to achieve excellence in healthcare delivery. They are a starting point, beginning with a mission that identifies why the organization exists, and ending with superior performance achievements based on well-defined business expectations that are transparent throughout an organization. But to fully achieve excellence in healthcare settings, healthcare teams need to integrate high-reliability characteristics into excellence pursuits. Why are high-reliability traits important to achieving consistent organizational outcomes?

High-reliability organizations (HROs) are organizations that operate in complex, high-hazard domains for extended periods without serious accidents or catastrophic failures. The concept of high reliability is attractive for health care because of the complexity of operations and the risk of significant and even potentially catastrophic consequences when failures occur in health care.[14]

> **High reliability in health care means consistent EXCELLENCE in quality and safety for every patient, EVERY TIME.**
>
> *—The Joint Commission Center for Transforming Healthcare*

HRO theory evolved from Normal Accident Theory work by Yale sociologist Charles Perrow. In 2001, Weick, Sutcliffe, and Obstfeld reconceptualized high-reliability theory to include collective mindfulness, a state whereby organizations pay collective attention to examine situations and outcomes. The researchers maintained that high-reliability organizations operate under challenging conditions yet experience fewer problems than would be anticipated because they have developed ways of "managing the unexpected" better than most organizations.[15] High reliability is a cultural mindset that prioritizes safety as a way of operating—all the time, every time. While standardization of structures, processes, and targeted outcomes can aid efforts to become an HRO, standardization without acculturation will prohibit achieving high-reliability outcomes in organizations. A high-reliability culture is infused with five core characteristics that drive organizational mindsets. (See Table 1.4 for characteristics of HROs.)

HROs are constantly evolving, responding to changes in the healthcare environment— HROs are a work in progress with teams who accept that no process is perfect and that there is always room for improvement. HRO theory is a way of thinking about situations and outcomes, then acting upon findings. Because each organization has unique needs and starting points, a cookbook approach cannot be used to acculturate organizations into HRO traits. To truly achieve HRO status, design and implementation processes required to acculturate organizations must be customized to an organization, the organization must be given time to adapt, and resources to educate and communicate progress must be available.

TABLE 1.4
CHARACTERISTICS OF HIGH-RELIABILITY ORGANIZATIONS (HROS)

CHARACTERISTIC	DESCRIPTION
Preoccupation with Failure	Everyone is aware of and thinking about the potential for failure. People understand that new threats emerge regularly from situations that no one imagined could occur, so all personnel actively think about what could go wrong and are alert to small signs of potential problems. The absence of errors or accidents leads not to complacency but to a heightened sense of vigilance for the next possible failure. Near misses are viewed as opportunities to learn about systems issues and potential improvements, rather than as evidence of safety.
Reluctance to Simplify	People resist simplifying their understanding of work processes and how and why things succeed or fail in their environment. People in HROs understand that the work is complex and dynamic. They seek underlying rather than surface explanations. While HROs recognize the value of standardization of workflows to reduce variation, they also appreciate the complexity inherent in the number of teams, processes, and relationships involved in conducting daily operations.
Sensitivity to Operations	Based on their understanding of operational complexity, people in HROs strive to maintain a high awareness of operational conditions. This sensitivity is often referred to as "big picture understanding" or "situation awareness." It means that people cultivate an understanding of the context of the current state of their work in relation to the unit or organizational state—i.e., what is going on around them—and how the current state might support or threaten safety.
Deference to Expertise	People in HROs appreciate that the people closest to the work are the most knowledgeable about the work. Thus, people in HROs know that in a crisis or emergency the person with greatest knowledge of the situation might not be the person with the highest status and seniority. Deference to local and situation expertise results in a spirit of inquiry and de-emphasis on hierarchy in favor of learning as much as possible about potential safety threats. In an HRO, everyone is expected to share concerns with others and the organizational climate is such that all staff members are comfortable speaking up about potential safety problems.
Commitment to Resilience	Commitment to resilience is rooted in the fundamental understanding of the frequently unpredictable nature of system failures. People in HROs assume the system is at risk for failure, and they practice performing rapid assessments of and responses to challenging situations. Teams cultivate situation assessment and cross monitoring so they may identify potential safety threats quickly and either respond before safety problems cause harm or mitigate the seriousness of the safety event.

Table from AHRQ PSNET. Retrtieved at https://psnet.ahrq.gov/primers/primer/31/high-reliabilityAHRQ

Sources: Weick, K. E., & Sutcliffe, K. M. (2015). *Managing the unexpected: Sustained performance in a complex world* (3rd ed.). San Francisco: John Wiley and Sons.

Hines, S., Luna, K., Lofthus, J. Marquardt, M., & Stelmokas, D. (2008, February). *Becoming a high reliability organization: Operational advice for hospital leaders.* AHRQ publication no. 08-0022. Rockville, MD: Agency for Healthcare Research and Quality.

Chassin, M. R., & Loeb, J. M. (2013). High-reliability health care: Getting there from here. *Milbank Quarterly,* 91(3): 459–490.

Rochlin, G. I. (1999). Safe operation as a social construct. *Ergonomics,* 42(11): 1549–1560.

Commitment from healthcare team members to embrace an HRO mindset is essential to delivering exceptional healthcare.

There are many factors that contribute to creating a culture of safety in an organization. As you embark on your excellence journey there are resources available to help you navigate cultural, regulatory, and evidence-based practices that will enable you to become a high-reliability organization.

Driving Forces for Culture of Safety

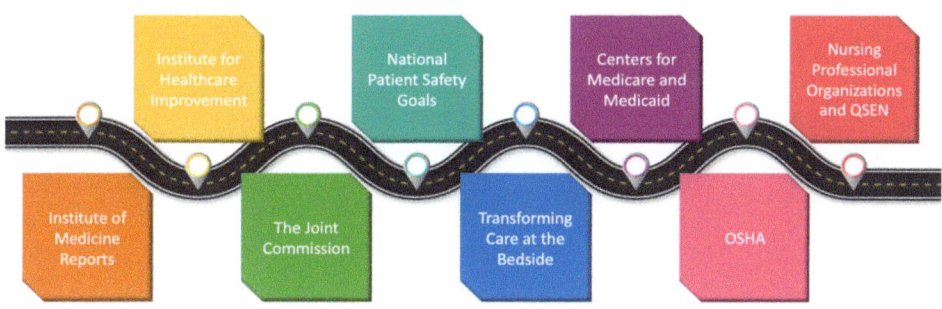

WHAT IS NURSING EXCELLENCE?

"As nurses are the largest component of the health care workforce and are also strongly involved in the detection and prevention of errors and adverse events, they and their work environment are critical elements of stronger patient safety defenses."

—Keeping Patients Safe: Transforming the Work Environment of Nurses (2004)

The IOM's groundbreaking report, *The Future of Nursing: Leading Change, Advancing Health*,[16] calls the profession of nursing to action to help fulfill the Patient Protection and Affordable Care Act (ACA) quality and cost-of-care goals. Healthcare spending is projected to rise from 17.4% of GDP in 2013 to 19.6% of GDP by 2024, equaling $5.4 trillion, with the government-sponsored share of health spending rising to 47% of 2024 national health expenditures, significantly driven by ACA coverage expansion, rising healthcare costs, and population aging.[17,18] To contain annual growth increases, interprofessional teams will need to work together to deliver new and improved care at a lower cost. Excellence in the provision of nursing care can serve as a leverage point to deliver higher-quality and lower-cost patient care in all delivery settings.

The nursing profession can and does make a difference: nurses have direct impact on patient care across the continuum of care delivery. Nursing is the largest segment of the U.S. healthcare workforce, with about 60% of nurses working in hospital settings and representing approximately 30% of inpatient labor costs.[16,19] Nurses provide a significant and large role in the delivery of health care. Dr. Stephanie Ferguson gets to the point: "Empowered nurses equal effective healthcare."[20]

We know that nursing practice directly impacts patient care, but how do we define healthcare excellence and the specific nursing and interprofessional practices needed to achieve it?

ANCC FRAMEWORK FOR HEALTH CARE EXCELLENCE

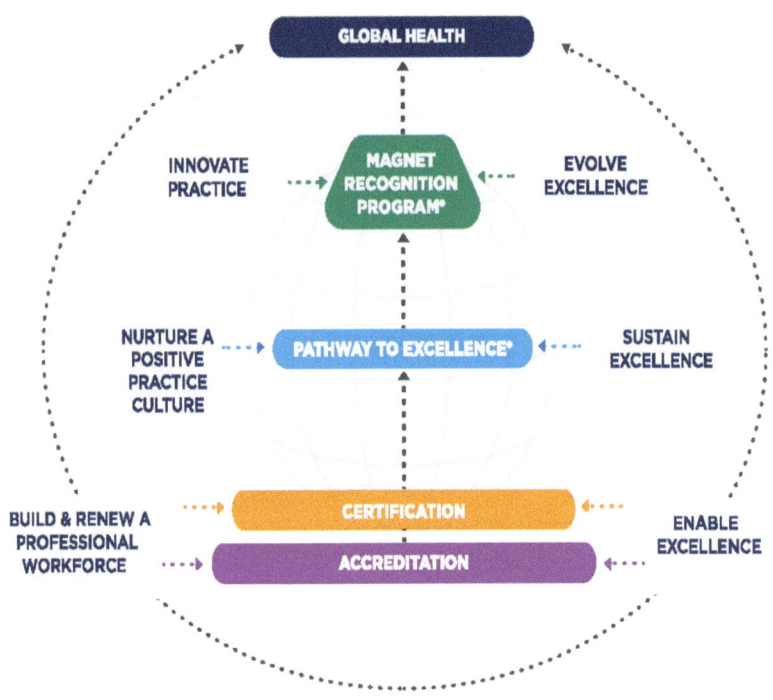

The American Nurses Credentialing Center (ANCC) has established global health standards promoting evidence-based nurse recognition programs that support the design, development, and implementation of nursing and interprofessional excellence outcomes. Accreditation standards offer guideposts on creating nurse and interprofessional continuing education programs, nurse transition into practice programs, and interprofessional accreditation standards. Certification exams used to assess specialized nursing competencies address how individuals can achieve personal excellence in the delivery of health care.

The IOM report *The Future of Nursing: Leading Change, Advancing Health* described nursing excellence as organizations that were "Magnets or Magnet-like." About 8% of US healthcare delivery systems achieve Magnet recognition, but there are also organizations that exhibit "Magnet-like" characteristics that lead to the delivery of quality patient care. Magnet-like organizations can use the Magnet model or other models to achieve excellence in patient care outcomes. Examples of models that promote nursing excellence include IOM's model of core competencies for health professionals,[21] AACN's Synergy Model for Patient Care®,[22] IHI's Always Events® model,[23] and QSEN's competencies for nursing.[24] (See Table 1.5 for information about the competency model components for these programs.) The models support components included in ANCC's Magnet Recognition Program® evaluation criteria but do not cover the full scope of what the Magnet Model offers to guide organizations toward nursing excellence.

TABLE 1.5
EXAMPLES OF MODELS SUPPORTING NURSING EXCELLENCE

MODEL	COMPETENCY MODEL COMPONENTS				
ANCC Magnet® Model	Provide patient-centered care	Participate in interdisciplinary teamwork	Use evidence-based practice	Apply quality improvement and nursing research	Capability to use informatics/ data in decision-making
IOM Core Competencies[21]	Provide patient-centered care	Participate in interdisciplinary teamwork	Use evidence-based practice	Apply quality improvement	Capability to use informatics
QSEN Competencies[24]	Patient-centered care	Teamwork and collaboration	Evidence-based practice	Quality improvement and safety	Informatics
AACN Synergy Model for Patient Care®[22]	A conceptual model of patient care for designing nursing practice and competencies required to care for critically ill patients. The model recognizes three levels of outcomes derived from the patient, nurse, and healthcare system. According to AACN, the basic premise of the model is that "optimal outcomes result from the synergy of a nurse's competencies matching the needs of patients and their families."[22]				
	Advocacy/ Moral Agency Response to Diversity Facilitation of Learning	Collaboration	Clinical Judgment Clinical Inquiry	Caring Practices Systems Thinking	Not specifically addressed in the model but expressed in the Clinical Inquiry Competency
IHI Always Events®[23]	A program that "recognizes the translation of person- and family-centered principles into tangible action by implementing innovative programs to enhance communication and collaboration with patients and families."[23] Now led by the Institute for Healthcare Improvement (IHI), defines Always Events® as "those aspects of care experience that should always occur when patients, their family members or other care partners, and service users interact with health care professionals and the health care delivery system."				

ANCC's Magnet Recognition Program® is the highest organizational credential for nursing excellence and the leading source of successful nursing practices and strategies worldwide. The Magnet Model is based on Donabedian's widely used 1966 conceptual model of structure, process, and outcomes that provides a framework for examining healthcare practices and evaluating quality. ANCC's Magnet Model is organized around five components: Transformational Leadership; Structural Empowerment; Exemplary Professional Practice; New Knowledge, Innovations, and Improvements; and Empirical Outcomes. The Magnet Model has been extensively researched, with the preponderance of research findings supporting the model criteria and outcomes.[25]

ANCC's Magnet® Model

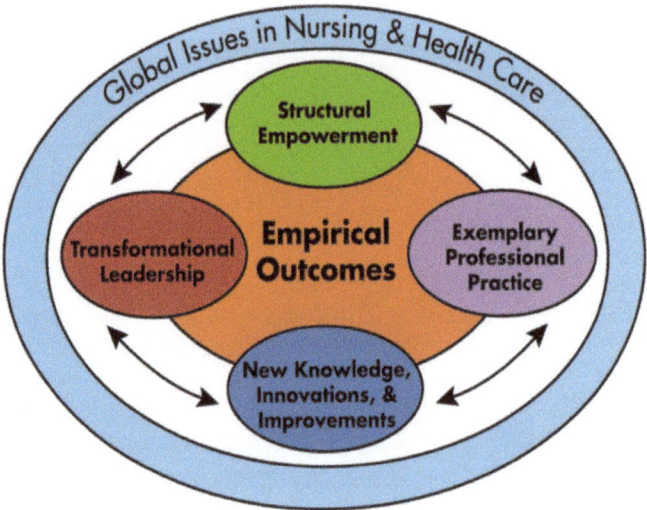

The Magnet Model is not prescriptive. The model provides opportunities for nursing organizations to innovate based on local healthcare delivery needs, organizational culture, and available resources within the healthcare system. There is not a "one size fits all" approach to fulfilling Magnet Recognition Program® criteria; original initiatives such as the Culture of Nursing Excellence (CONE),[26] Loyola University Medical Center's Nursing Excellence Award Program,[27] Saint Joseph's Hospital of Atlanta clinical ladder redesign, and Catawba Valley Medical Center's leadership safety huddle[28] are examples of innovative approaches to achieving quality care through the Magnet Recognition Program® model. Table 1.4 summarizes excellence approaches.

The updated 2019 Magnet® Application Manual defines terms associated with interprofessional collaborative practice (IPCP) and identifies specific standards related to IPCP.

Investigate further the Magnet® Model components by accessing the Magnet Model overview at https://www.nursingworld.org/organizational-programs /magnet/magnet-model/ and consider which components your organization would excel in and those that would provide challenges.

Review Linda Aiken's Overview of State of Research: Organizational Credentialing presentation at http://iom.nationalacademies.org/~/media/Files /Activity%20Files/Workforce/NursingCredentialing/2013-JAN-14/Linda%20 Aiken.pdf.

WORKSHEET

Discovering Magnet Model Opportunities and Challenges

Instructions: Access ANCC's Magnet Recognition Program® at https://www .nursingworld.org/organizational-programs/magnet/magnet-model/.

For each model component listed below, identify characteristics that define the domain.

Evaluate whether your organization is ready to integrate the Magnet Model sources of evidence into structures, processes, and outcome measures currently supporting your organization.

MODEL COMPONENT	KEY CHARACTERISTICS	YOUR READINESS
Transformational Leadership Notes:		o Yes o No
Structural Empowerment Notes:		o Yes o No
Exemplary Professional Practice Notes:		o Yes o No
New Knowledge, Innovations, and Improvements Notes:		o Yes o No
Empirical Outcomes Notes:		o Yes o No

For example, a Magnet Exemplary Professional Practice standard requires organizations to have clearly delineated policies or management practices that address interprofessional conflict. Standards for meeting Transformational Leadership evidence include documentation of organizational change initiatives that encompass nursing working with other departments across the organization. Structural Empowerment standards specify that clinical nurses are involved in interprofessional decision-making groups across the organization. Magnet standards require an example of interprofessional group activity that influenced the clinical care of patients. The standards seek to align IPCP endeavors with patient care impacts.

HOW DOES THE MAGNET MODEL COMPARE WITH OTHER ORGANIZATIONAL QUALITY PROGRAMS?

Porter and Tanner describe business or organizational excellence as a continuous process of improvement that requires:

- Engaged people to transform the organization,

- Measurements based on a clear understanding of what performance is expected,

- Assessments integrated as part of the learning process,

- Identification of strengths and improvement opportunities, and

- Systematic tracking of progress and review of organizational activities and results compared to a defined excellence model.

Porter and Tanner's work on assessing organizational excellence provides a way to compare and contrast the Magnet Recognition Program® model to other quality frameworks. Programs such as Total Quality Management (TQM), ISO9000, Business Process Re-engineering (BPR), Six Sigma[SM], the Deming Prize, and the Malcolm Baldrige Quality Award are included in their organizational excellence framework review. The researchers conclude that such award frameworks serve a purpose to help organizations implement best practices for excellence strategies, assessments, and benchmarking that can lead to improved organizational performance.[29] They found that most of the organizational excellence frameworks share common criteria and require organizations to integrate improvement criteria into organizational structures and processes. Table 1.6 details Porter and Tanner's core themes of organizational excellence across the quality frameworks.

ANCC's Magnet Model provides a roadmap to achieve nursing excellence using five model components and sources of evidence to drive organizational performance focused on improving the quality of patient care while lowering costs. The Magnet Model is congruent with other nursing and organizational excellence programs, offering a comprehensive approach aimed toward improving patient care, nurse safety, nurse satisfaction and retention, shared decision-making, and interprofessional collaboration. The Magnet Recognition Program® is often cited as the "gold standard" in achieving nursing excellence.

TABLE 1.6
PORTER AND TANNER'S COMMON CRITERIA ACROSS ORGANIZATIONAL EXCELLENCE FRAMEWORKS[29]

THEME	DEFINITION
Leadership	Establish a clear direction and values Maintain a customer focus Empower employees
Customer Focus	Pay attention to customer feedback Consider current and prospective customers' needs Focus on customer loyalty and retention Design processes that best serve the customer
Strategic Alignment	Focus on strategy development, implementation tactics, and alignment within the organization
Organizational Learning, Innovation, and Continuous Improvement	Design sharing of knowledge processes and values Focus on continuous learning and feedback processes and implement enhancements
People	Develop shared values Create a culture of trust and empowerment
Mutually Beneficial Relationships	Seek out external partners to form synergistic relationships that benefit both partners Deliver continual value to partners such as strategy sharing, cost sharing on projects, advisory boards, etc.
Manage by Facts	Collect facts to systematically manage processes Gain customer feedback and act on it Evaluate processes and engage in continuous improvement
Expected Results	Create value for all key stakeholders—measure outcomes (quantitative and qualitative)
Social Responsibility	Model ethical behavior and good citizenship

EXERCISE 1.4
COMPARING HIGH RELIABILITY ORGANIZATION TRAITS WITH PORTER AND TANNER'S EXCELLENCE FRAMEWORK

Compare Table 1.4, HRO traits, with Table 1.6, Porter and Tanner's themes.

a. How are the traits and themes similar?

b. How do they differ?

Compare Porter and Tanner's common quality framework provided in Table 1.6 with your organizational excellence framework.

- How does your current excellence framework align with Porter and Tanner's common quality framework?

Compare the HRO framework provided in Table 1.4 with your organizational excellence framework.

- How does your current excellence framework align with the High Reliability Organization framework?

Compare the Magnet Model framework in Exercise 1.3 with your organizational excellence framework.

- How does your current excellence framework align with the Magnet Model framework?

Scan the Fundamentals of Magnet® Gap Analysis Tool located in Step 7: Tools and Resources (pg. 173).

The gap analysis tool provides an overview of ACA components and how they can be considered in an organizational excellence model. The tool in Step 7 is not related to nor endorsed by the Magnet Recognition Program. For official ANCC tools available to support organizations interested in the Magnet Program, see: https://www.nursingworld.org/nurses-books/magnet -organizational-self-assessment/

- How is your organization currently meeting ACA and excellence standards?

List existing or proposed quality models supporting your organization.

- What models best support your excellence goals?
- What additional value do you think the Magnet Recognition Program® can provide to your organization and to your customers?

HOW DOES YOUR WORK ENVIRONMENT MEASURE UP?

ANCC's Pathway to Excellence® Program recognizes organizations committed to achieving a positive practice environment with an engaged workforce. The program provides a
framework for creating an ideal work environment that fosters workplace satisfaction and
provider well-being. Congruent with Magnet Program standards, the 2016 Pathway to
Excellence® standards include an emphasis on interprofessional collaboration and promoting a culture of health in communities. Research suggests that healthy work environments
improve nurse satisfaction, patient satisfaction, and the quality of care. Table 1.7 lists the six
focus areas in the Pathway to Excellence® that are designed to achieve a positive practice
environment.

TABLE 1.7
PATHWAY TO EXCELLENCE® STANDARDS*

THEME	CONSTRUCTS SUPPORTING THEMES
Shared Decision-Making	Nurses control the practice of nursing with an established governance structure
	Ethics involving interprofessional collaboration
	Staff support during ethical concerns
	Direct-care nurse involvement in organizational decision-making
Leadership	CNO is qualified and participates in all levels of the organization
	Nurses in leadership roles are competent and accountable
	Actively engages staff in resource allocation, cost management, and advocacy
	Leadership development and succession planning
	Application of change management principles
	Staying current with issues and trends impacting direct care nurses
Safety	The work environment is safe and healthy
	Systems and measures are in place to protect patients, families, and nurses
	Safeguards for unforeseen events are in place
	Security measures against violence are readily available and known
	Policies are developed by interprofessional teams
	Nurse involvement in staffing decisions
	Interprofessional collaboration during care transitions
Quality	A quality program and evidence-based practice are used and measured with external and internal benchmarks
	Interprofessional collaboration for organization-wide initiatives
	Interprofessional collaboration to engage patients and families in making decisions about care
	Staff alignment with the mission, vision, and goals of the organization

THEME	CONSTRUCTS SUPPORTING THEMES
Well-Being	A balanced lifestyle is encouraged
	Flexible scheduling is accommodated as possible
	Equitable compensation is provided, and retention incentives are used
	Nurses are supported and recognized for achievements in community service, advocacy, and improvements to population health
	Staff's personal well-being is supported by initiatives both internal and external to workplace
	Health assessment for staff and initiatives to support results
	Improvement initiatives to improve population and community health
Professional Development	Orientation, including needs assessments, prepare nurses for the work environment
	Professional development and/or mentoring are/is provided and used
	Collaborative relationships are valued and supported
	Seamless transitions into practice programs are utilized.

Access to the Pathway to Excellence® Gap Analysis tool can be found at: https://www.nursingworld.org/organizational-programs/accreditation/ptap/resources/gap-analysis/

*Interprofessional collaboration is integrated in the standards. Access to the Pathway to Excellence® Gap Analysis tool can be found at: https://www.nursingworld.org/organizational-programs/accreditation/ptap/resources/gap-analysis/

Magnet and Pathway to Excellence® recognition programs each provide unique frameworks for organizations to infuse evidenced-based organizational excellence structures, processes, and outcome measurements into healthcare delivery decisions. Research suggests that by incorporating these standards into everyday operations, patients and healthcare teams benefit. Interprofessional collaboration standards have been added to both recognition programs to leverage the knowledge, skills, and abilities of all healthcare team members. Research shows that as interprofessional collaboration takes hold, patient safety and quality outcomes improve.[30]

ACCREDITATION-BUILDING OPPORTUNITIES FOR EXCELLENCE

ANCC's Accreditation program recognizes the need for high-quality continuing nursing education (CNE), interprofessional continuing education (IPCE), transition-to-practice programs, and skills-based competency programs. Around the world, ANCC-accredited organizations provide nurses with the knowledge and skills to help improve care and patient outcomes.

The accreditation CNE model is based on Donabedian's framework of structure, process, and outcome measures as shown in Exhibit 1.6.

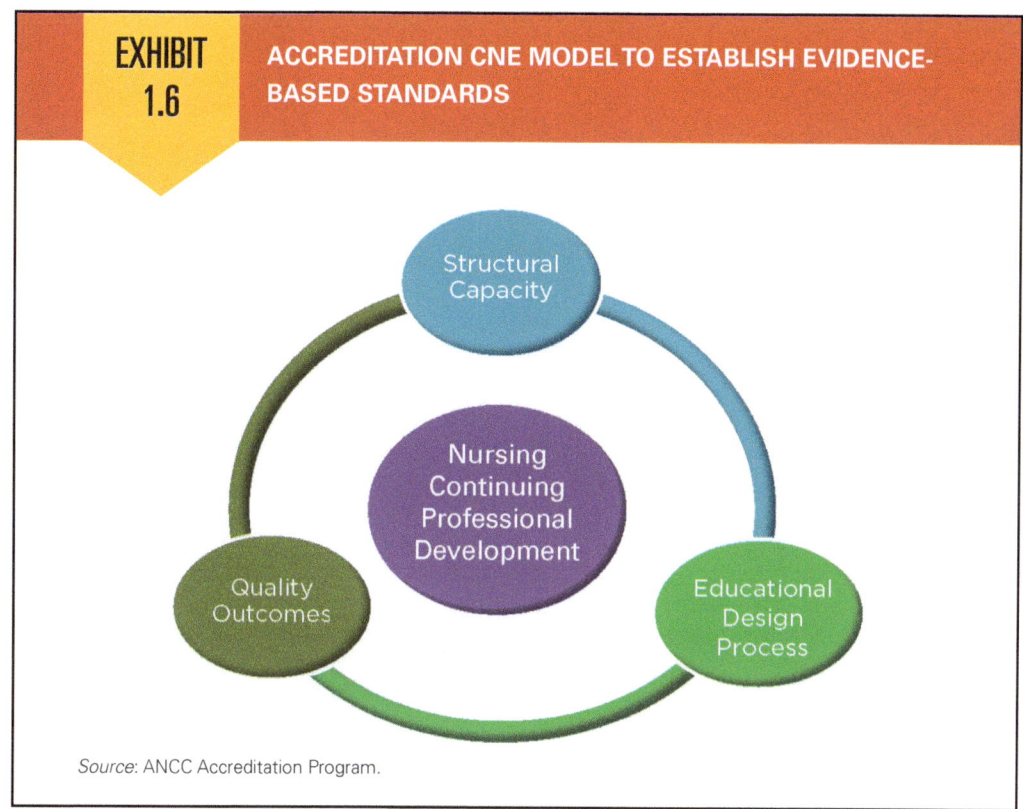

EXHIBIT 1.6 ACCREDITATION CNE MODEL TO ESTABLISH EVIDENCE-BASED STANDARDS

Structural Capacity

Nursing Continuing Professional Development

Quality Outcomes

Educational Design Process

Source: ANCC Accreditation Program.

Nursing continuing professional development (NCPD) standards use evidence-based criteria to plan, implement, and evaluate the quality of NCPD activities. Recognizing that organizations often create education programs serving interprofessional healthcare teams, ANCC teamed with the Accreditation Council for Continuing Medical Education (ACCME) and the Accreditation Council for Pharmacy Education (ACPE) to create an innovative Joint Accreditation™ for Interprofessional Continuing Education program. Transition-to-practice programs (TPP) are another system employed by organizations to support competent professional practice. These programs are designed to support newly licensed RN progression from education to practice as they move from student to professional, nurses transitioning between practice settings, and APRNs entering practice. The National Council of State Boards of Nursing (NCSBN) and the American Association of Colleges of Nursing (AACN) have defined TPPs as a formal program of active learning that includes a series of educational sessions and work experiences for newly licensed RNs.

ANCC'S Practice Transition Accreditation Program (PTAP) is based on evidence collected through peer-reviewed research (see Table 1.8 for research examples). The PTAP program supports practice transitions for RN Residencies, RN Fellowships, and APRN Fellowships. The model is based on Benner's Novice to Expert framework applied to six domains that have shown to be critical to achieve effective transitions in work environments.

The six domains identified to prepare teams for effective transitions are provided in Exhibit 1.7.

TABLE 1.8
TRANSITION INTO PRACTICE SUPPORTING RESEARCH

BENEFITS	EVIDENCE
Reduced turnover/increased retention	Goode, C. J., Reid Ponte, P., & Sullivan Havens, D. (2016). Residency for transition into practice. *Journal of Nursing Administration, 46*(2), 82–86. Ulrich, B., Krozek, C., Early, S., Ashlock, C. H., Africa, L. M., & Carman, M. L. (2010). Improving retention, confidence, and competence of new graduate nurses: Results from a 10-year longitudinal database. *Nursing Economics, 28*(6), 363–375.
Increases in skill confidence, ability to organize and prioritize work; improved comfort communicating with team members, patients, and families; and stronger unit clinical leadership	Goode, C. J., Lynn, M. R., Krsek, C., & Bednash, G. D. (2009). Nurse residency programs: An essential requirement for nursing. *Journal of Nursing Administration, 27*(3), 142–147.
Residency programs emphasizing collaboration across disciplines has been found to enhance a positive learning environment.	Anderson, G., Hair, C., & Todero, C. (2012). Nurse residency programs: An evidence-based review of theory, process and outcomes. *Journal of Professional Nursing, 28*(4), 203–212.

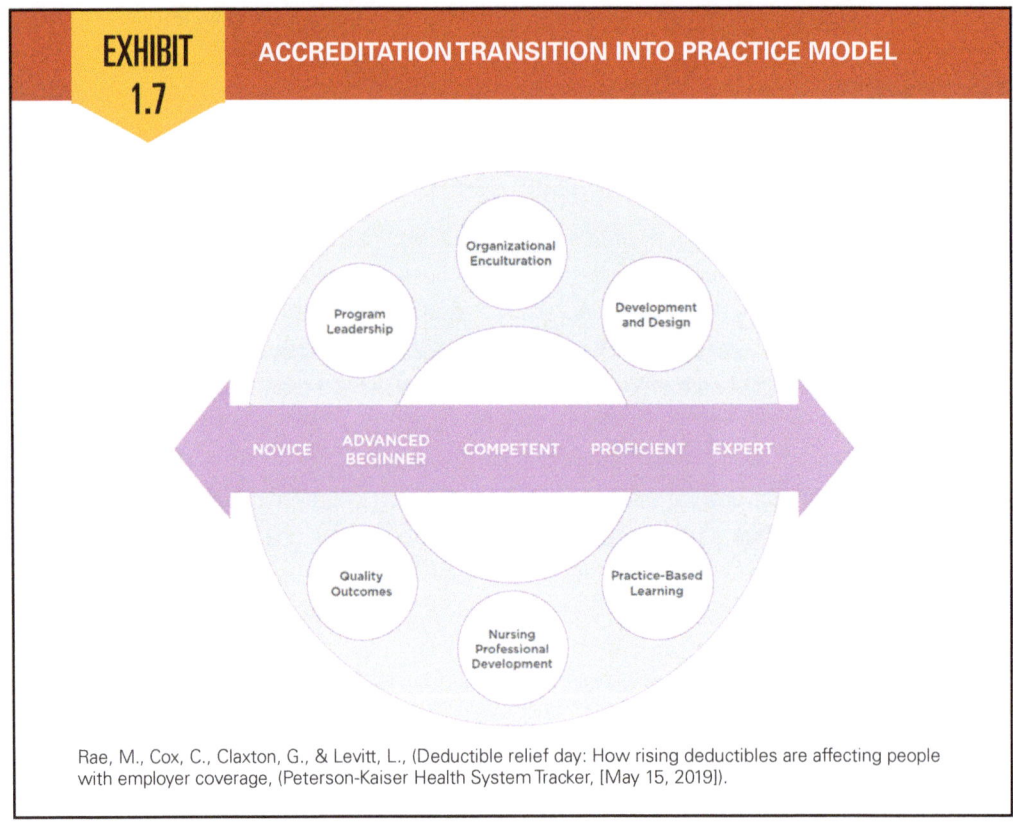

EXHIBIT 1.7

ACCREDITATION TRANSITION INTO PRACTICE MODEL

Rae, M., Cox, C., Claxton, G., & Levitt, L., (Deductible relief day: How rising deductibles are affecting people with employer coverage, (Peterson-Kaiser Health System Tracker, [May 15, 2019]).

To support efforts in creating PTAP programs within organizations, free templates to gauge your organization's baseline readiness can be downloaded at https://www.nursingworld.org/organizational-programs/accreditation/ptap/download-ptap-manual/.

Resource Links

TABLE 1.9
NAVIGATING MEASURES: RESOURCES TO GET YOU STARTED

RESOURCE	SOURCE
ANCC Accreditation Programs	https://www.nursingworld.org/organizational-programs/accreditation/ http://www.jointaccreditation.org
CMS Quality Payment Program	https://qpp.cms.gov/about/resource-library
CMS Meaningful Measures Framework and HUB	https://www.cms.gov/Medicare/Quality-Initiatives-Patient-Assessment-Instruments/QualityInitiativesGenInfo/CMS-Quality-Strategy.html
Institute for Healthcare Improvement (IHI)	http://www.ihi.org
Magnet Recognition Program®	https://www.nursingworld.org/organizational-programs/magnet/
NQF Nurse Sensitive Indicators: National Voluntary Consensus Standards for Nursing-Sensitive Care: An Initial Performance Measure Set	http://www.qualityforum.org/Projects/n-r/Nursing-Sensitive_Care_Initial_Measures/Nursing_Sensitive_Care__Initial_Measures.aspx
Pathway to Excellence® Program	https://www.nursingworld.org/organizational-programs/pathway/
Quality Improvement Organizations (QIOs)	http://www.qioprogram.org/
QSEN Competencies	http://qsen.org/competencies/

INTERPROFESSIONAL COLLABORATIVE PRACTICE (IPCP)—A STEP TOWARD EXCELLENCE

In 2010, the Institute of Medicine (IOM) recommended that nurses be educated with physicians and other health professionals through their initial training and during their careers.[30] According to the World Health Organization, interprofessional collaborative practice happens "when multiple health workers from different professional backgrounds work together with patients, families, carers [sic], and communities to deliver the highest quality of care."[31] Why pursue IPCP in your organization? Because research demonstrates that effective interprofessional teams provide safer and higher quality patient care.[30]

The Affordable Care Act supported pilot projects to experiment with the development and implementation of IPCP initiatives. Since 2010, grant organizations such as the Robert Wood Johnson Foundation, Josiah Macy Jr. Foundation, and the Doctor's Company Foundation have supported pilot projects that explore new working models for interprofessional collaborative practice. Voluntary recognition and accreditation programs such as ANCC's now include interprofessional collaborative practice standards.

Interprofessional education standards include interprofessional collaborative practice in education curriculums. Accreditors for healthcare professions such as the American Association of Medical Colleges (AAMC), the Commission on Collegiate Nursing Education (CCNE), and the Accreditation Review Commission on Education for the Physician Assistant (ARC-PA), now require educational curriculums to include IPCP content, and programs must demonstrate activities related to interprofessional, patient-centered teams. AAMC survey data highlights 2017–2018 curriculum goals focused on the development of IPCP competencies. Of significant note are the top two, which target understanding roles and team skills. This aligns with research findings suggesting these areas remain barriers to successfully implement interprofessional collaborative teams. (See Exhibit 1.8.)

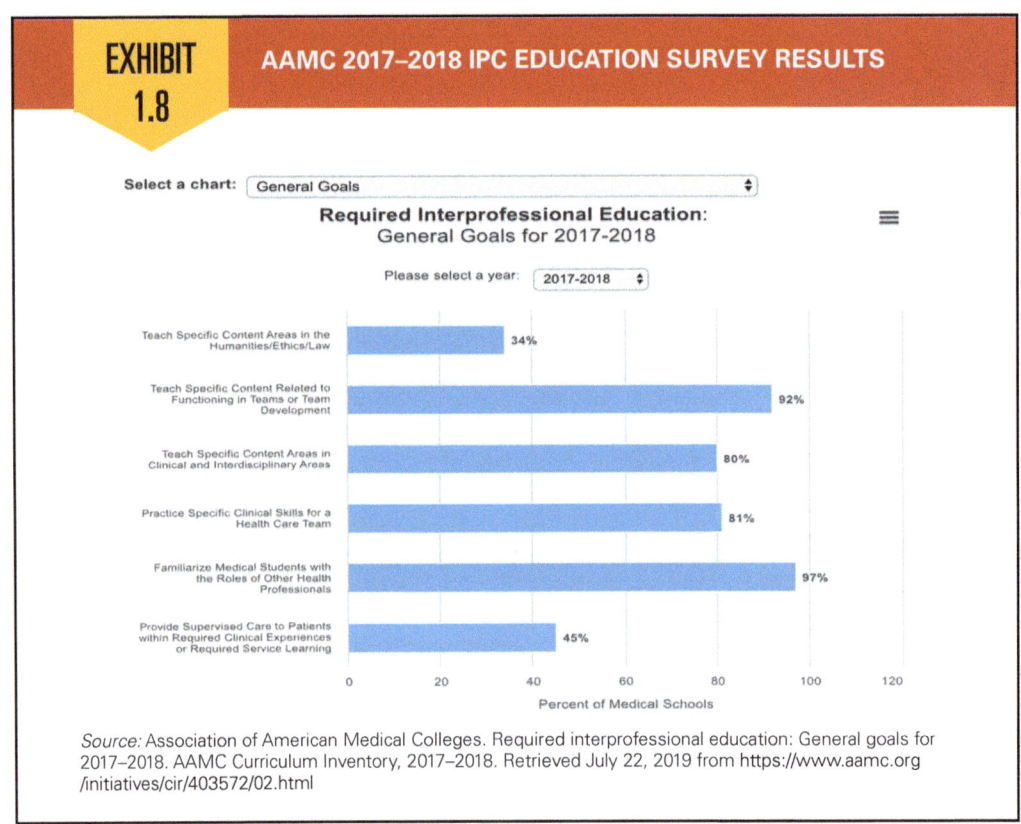

EXHIBIT 1.8

AAMC 2017–2018 IPC EDUCATION SURVEY RESULTS

Select a chart: General Goals

Required Interprofessional Education: General Goals for 2017-2018

Please select a year: 2017-2018

Goal	Percent of Medical Schools
Teach Specific Content Areas in the Humanities/Ethics/Law	34%
Teach Specific Content Related to Functioning in Teams or Team Development	92%
Teach Specific Content Areas in Clinical and Interdisciplinary Areas	80%
Practice Specific Clinical Skills for a Health Care Team	81%
Familiarize Medical Students with the Roles of Other Health Professionals	97%
Provide Supervised Care to Patients within Required Clinical Experiences or Required Service Learning	45%

Percent of Medical Schools

Source: Association of American Medical Colleges. Required interprofessional education: General goals for 2017–2018. AAMC Curriculum Inventory, 2017–2018. Retrieved July 22, 2019 from https://www.aamc.org/initiatives/cir/403572/02.html

While benefits of IPCP are well documented, organizations remain challenged to fully implement IPCP programs. Barriers to IPCP team success at the organizational level include cultural norms concerning team roles, lack of appreciation of other healthcare team member skills, teams with minimal experience in team building, legal issues regarding scope-of-practice concerns, financial reimbursement and regulatory constraints, and hierarchical structures that discourage interprofessional collaboration.

Interprofessional collaborative practice can succeed if organizations commit to implementing IPCP competencies that are supplemented with real-world interprofessional team experiences. Lessons learned from a unique and successful pilot, *Interprofessional Longitudinal Clinical Experience (ILCE)*, with Yale University's School of Nursing, School of Medicine, and Physician Associate Program provide insights about the design and implementation of successful IPCP teams. While the Yale project took place in an educational healthcare setting to assist master's and doctoral level students to develop new IPCP competencies, lessons learned from the pilot can provide guideposts for organizations seeking to implement IPCP teams.[32]

The Yale team leading the IPCP pilots functioned as equal partners across nursing, medicine, and physician assistant programs. Over a four-year period three pilot studies were completed, with each pilot program benefiting from lessons learned to continually improve the IPCP model. Interviews with two of the program leaders, Dr. Eve Colson and Dr. Linda Honan, reiterated their research findings—designing and implementing an interprofessional collaborative education program is hard work, it requires room to fail, it can be frustrating, not everyone embraces the cultural changes needed to implement teams, and IPCP teams must have ambassadors who support the change management initiatives required to alter structures, processes, and cultures.

Extrapolating from the Yale ILCE pilot research, here are suggestions for organizations seeking to implement IPCP teams:

- Interprofessional collaborative teams need role models who project equality among healthcare professions. IPCP governance decisions serve as a megaphone about cultural expectations, so be clear about where you want to lead others and how you will lead them.

- Culture is key—long-held norms of hierarchies and roles will be altered. Be prepared to implement change management initiatives. Identify your cultural ambassadors and recruit HR and organizational design expertise to help with organizational change.

- Start small. Select a topic or patient domain that can be tested with a small team of volunteers interested in promulgating interprofessional practices. Recruit enthusiasts.

- Seek feedback about the initiative and adjust accordingly. Identify pros/cons and be transparent about where you are and where you are headed. As the Yale pilot found, you need a thick skin.

- Don't give up when it gets rough—and it will! Stay the course and encourage honest participation from those who will be truth-tellers.

The pursuit of excellence is a crooked path that is a unique journey for every organization. Step 1 highlighted elements of what excellence is, identified key drivers impacting excellence, and presented models that can help your organization excel. Step 2 takes you into the world of interprofessional collaborative practice so you can begin to identify cultural priorities and competencies that will accelerate your journey toward becoming a high-reliability organization.

REFERENCES

1. Division for Sustainable Development. (2015). *Transforming our world: the 2030 Agenda for Sustainable Development.* New York: The General Assembly. Retrieved from https://sustainabledevelopment.un.org/post2015/transformingourworld. Graphics retrieved from https://sustainabledevelopment.un.org/sdgs

2. Delivering quality health services: a global imperative for universal health coverage. Geneva: World Health Organization, Organization for Economic Co-operation and Development, and The World Bank; 2018. Licence: CC BY-NC-SA 3.0 IGO. Retrieved from https://read.oecd-ilibrary.org/social-issues-migration-health/delivering-quality-health-services-a-global -imperative_9789264300309-en#page1

3. Institute of Medicine. (2001). *Crossing the quality chasm: A new health system for the 21st century.* Washington, DC: the National Academies Press; 2001 (https://doi.org/10.17226/10027)

4. Six Domains of Health Care Quality. Content last reviewed November 2018. Agency for Healthcare Research and Quality, Rockville, MD. http://www.ahrq.gov/talkingquality/measures/six-domains.html

5. Operating Plan for Fiscal Year 2019. Content last reviewed November 2018. Agency for Healthcare Research and Quality, Rockville, MD. Retrieved from http://www.ahrq.gov/cpi/about/mission/operating-plan/index.html

6. Kohn, L. T., Corrigan, J. M., & Donaldson, M. S. (Eds.); Committee on Quality and Health Care in America, Institute of Medicine. (1999). *To err is human: Building a safer health system.* Washington, DC: National Academies Press. Retrieved from http://www.nap.edu/openbook.php?record_id=9728&page=R1

7. Center for Clinical Standards and Quality, Centers for Medicare & Medicaid Services. (2015). 2015 National impact assessment of the Centers for Medicare & Medicaid Services (CMS) quality measures report. Baltimore: Author. Retrieved from https://www.cms.gov/Medicare/Quality-Initiatives-Patient-Assessment-Instruments/QualityMeasures/Quality MeasurementImpactReports.html

8. 2018 National Impact Assessment of the Centers for Medicare & Medicaid Services (CMS) Quality Measures Report. Baltimore, MD: US Department of Health and Human Services, Centers for Medicare & Medicaid Services; February 28, 2018. Available at: https://www.cms.gov/Medicare/Quality-Initiatives-Patient-Assessment-Instruments/QualityMeasures /National-Impact-Assessment-of-the-Centers-for-Medicare-and-Medicaid-Services-CMS-Quality-Measures-Reports.html

9. Rae, M., Copeland, R., Cox, C. & Kaiser Family Foundation, Tracking the rise in premium contributions and cost-sharing for families with large employer coverage, (Peterson-Kaiser Health System Tracker, [August 14, 2019]) . Accessed at https:// www.healthsystemtracker.org/?sfid=4356&_sft_category=access-affordability,health-well-being,spending,quality-of-care

10. United Health Foundation. America's Health Rankings 2018 Annual Report. Accessed at https://www.americashealth rankings.org/

11. Rae, M., Cox, C., Claxton, G., & Levitt, L. Deductible relief day: How rising deductibles are affecting people with employer coverage. (2019). Kaiser Family Foundation briefs (Peterson-Kaiser Health System Tracker, [May 15, 2019]). Retrieved from https://www.healthsystemtracker.org/brief/deductible-relief-day-how-rising-deductibles-are-affecting-people-with -employer-coverage/#

12. Robert Pear, "Hospitals Must Now Post Prices. But it May Take a Brain Surgeon to Decipher Them," *New York Times*, January 13, 2019, https://www.nytimes.com/2019/01/13/us/politics/hospital-prices-online.html

13. American Society for Quality. What is organizational excellence? Milwaukee, WI. Accessed at https://asq.org/quality -resources/organizational-excellence

14. Hines S, Luna, K, Lofthus J, et al. Becoming a High Reliability Organization: Operational Advice for Hospital Leaders. (Prepared by the Lewin Group under Contract No. 290-04-0011.) AHRQ Publication No. 08-0022. Rockville, MD: Agency for Healthcare Research and Quality. April 2008.

15. AHRQ. Patient Safety Primer: High Reliability. Washington, DC: US Department of Health and Human Services, Agency for Health Care Research and Quality. January 2019. Retrieved at https://psnet.ahrq.gov/primers/primer/31/high-reliability

16. Institute of Medicine. (2011). *The future of nursing: Leading change, advancing health.* Washington, DC: National Academies Press.

17. Keehan, S. P., Cuckler, G. A., Sisko, A. M., Madison, A. J., Smith, S. D. Stone, D. A., ... Lizonitz, J. M. (2015). National health expenditure projection, 2014–24: Spending growth faster than recent trends. *Health Affairs*, 34(8),1407–1417.

18. Centers for Medicare & Medicaid Services. National health expenditure data: Projected. Retrieved from https://www .cms.gov/Research-Statistics-Data-and-Systems/Statistics-Trends-and-Reports/NationalHealthExpendData /NationalHealthAccountsProjected.html

19. The KPMG Healthcare & Pharmaceutical Institute. (2011). KPMG's 2011 U.S. hospital nursing labor costs study. Retrieved from http://www.natho.org/pdfs/KPMG_2011_Nursing_LaborCostStudy.pdf

20. Ferguson, S. (2013). The global quest for nursing excellence. *Journal of Nursing Administration*, 43(11), 555–556.

21. Greiner, A. C., & Knebel, E. (Eds.). (2003). *Health professions education: A bridge to quality.* IOM Committee on the Health Professions Education Summit. Washington, DC: The National Academies Press.

22. Hardin, S. R., & Kaplow, R. (2005). *Synergy for clinical excellence: The AACN synergy model for patient care.* Burlington, MA: Jones & Bartlett.

23. Institute for Healthcare Improvement. (2012). Always events. Retrieved from http://www.ihi.org/Engage/Initiatives /PatientFamilyCenteredCare/Pages/AlwaysEvents.aspx

24. QSEN Institute. (2014). Competencies. Retrieved from http://qsen.org/competencies/

25. Aiken, L. H. (2013). Overview of state of research: Organizational credentialing. Retrieved from http://iom.national academies.org/~/media/Files/Activity%20Files/Workforce/NursingCredentialing/2013-JAN-14/Linda%20Aiken.pdf

26. Roberts-Turner, R., Coleman, L., Guanci, G., Kunze-Humbel, T., & Walczak, D. (2014). Creating and sustaining a clinical environment of nursing excellence. *Nursing Management*, 45(7), 48–52.

27. Jasovsky, D. A., Grant, V. A., Lang, M., Deveereus, B. F., Altier, M. E., Bird, S. R. Hindle, P. A. (2010). How do you define nursing excellence? *Nursing Management*, 41(10), 19–24.

28. Beard, E. L. Jr., & Sharkey, K. (2013). Innovation amidst radical cost containment in health care. *Nursing Administration Quarterly*, 37(2), 116–121.

29. Tanner, S., & Porter, L. (2004). *Assessing business excellence* (2nd ed.). Burlington, MA: Elsevier Butterworth Heinmann.

30. Robert Wood Johnson Foundation. What Can Be Done to Encourage More Interprofessional Collaboration in Health Care? Health Policy Snapshot: Workforce. Issue Brief. 2011. Retrieved from https://www.rwjf.org/en/library/research/2011/09/what-can-be-done-to-encourage-more-interprofessional-collaborati.html

31. World Health Organization. (2010). *Framework for Action on Interprofessional Education & Collaborative Practice.* WHO Press. Accessed at: http://whqlibdoc.who.int/hq/2010/WHO_HRH_HPN_10.3_eng.pdf?ua=1

32. Fahs, D.B., Honan, L., Gonzalez-Colaso, R., & Colson, E.R. (2017). Interprofessional education development: Not for the faint of heart. *Advances in Medical Education and Practice*, 8, 329–336.

INTERPROFESSIONAL COLLABORATIVE PRACTICE (IPCP) AND INTERPROFESSIONAL EDUCATION (IPE)

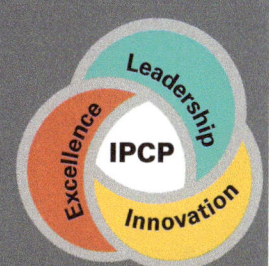

STEP

2

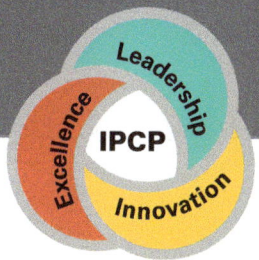

INTERPROFESSIONAL COLLABORATIVE PRACTICE (IPCP) AND INTERPROFESSIONAL EDUCATION (IPE)

As the evidence for IPE continues to evolve, we will develop greater knowledge of how it can most effectively be planned and implemented, and its relationship to developing collaborative competencies that can positively affect the delivery of patient care and health outcomes.

—Dr. Scott Reeves, IPE Expert

INTRODUCTION

Nursing excellence must be embedded within a framework of interprofessional collaborative practice (IPCP) to achieve organizational excellence, and nursing is well positioned to lead the transformation. From bedside to boardroom and hospital to home, nurses are integrated into every aspect of the healthcare delivery system. Nurses must be able to function both as members and as leaders of interprofessional healthcare teams and be able to quantify that contribution toward meeting organizational goals. This chapter provides an overview of IPCP including strategies that nursing leaders and others can implement to achieve success. Credentials such as those awarded to organizations (Magnet, Pathway, Accreditation), programs (Accreditation), and individuals (Certification) provide a framework as well as a validation mechanism of successful implementation.

RECOMMENDED RESOURCE

The National Center for Interprofessional Practice and Education provides tools and resources for interprofessional education and collaborative practice communities. See https://nexusipe.org/advancing/assessment-evaluation-start.

INTERPROFESSIONAL COLLABORATIVE PRACTICE

The World Health Organization (WHO) defines interprofessional collaborative practice (IPCP) as occurring "when multiple health workers from different professional backgrounds work together with patients, families, carers [sic], and communities to deliver the highest quality of care." This definition forms a framework for the core competencies of IPCP that have been widely endorsed and adopted by credentialing bodies in academic and practice settings.[1-4]

Goals of improving IPCP can be categorized into the domains of the Quadruple Aim: improve population health, improve the patient experience, reduce cost, and improve the work life of healthcare clinicians and staff.[5-6] When healthcare teams collaborate, patient outcomes can improve, and the overall patient experience is more satisfying. Collaboration can result in reduced waste and improve overall efficiency. And working in unison can create an environment of mutual trust, limit the demands on any one profession, reduce overall stress, and enhance overall job satisfaction.[7]

There are numerous examples of positive outcomes when the healthcare team practices collaboratively. Unfortunately, there are also devastating consequences when the healthcare team fails to work together. A systematic review published by Reeves and colleagues (2016) cited studies that explored the relationship between IPCE and practice change and patient outcomes.[8] Positive practice changes and patient outcomes cited in studies included improving service delivery across a range of areas such as illness prevention, patient screening, and referrals between agencies, safety practices, and clinical outcomes such as mortality rates, recorded clinical errors, or patient length of stay. The negative consequences attributed to team failures have also been noted, particularly in root cause analysis or failure analysis reports. The annual sentinel event reporting summary of the Joint Commission, for example, represents how errors in clinical practice can harm patients (https://www.jointcommission.org/sentinel_event.aspx).

The Robert Wood Johnson Foundation (RWJF) published a report of findings from a workshop describing how healthcare organizations promote interprofessional collaboration to advance a Culture of Health.[9] The report defined IPCP as follows:

> *Effective interprofessional collaboration promotes the active participation of each discipline in patient care, where all disciplines are working together and fully engaging patients and those who support them, and leadership on the team adapts based on patient needs.*

> *Effective interprofessional collaboration enhances patient and family-centered goals and values, provides mechanisms for continuous communication among caregivers, and optimizes participation in clinical*

decision-making within and across disciplines. It fosters respect for the disciplinary contributions of all professionals.

Twenty organizations representing diverse healthcare settings participated in the RWFJ workshop and collectively identified guiding principles required to create an environment of interprofessional collaboration. These principles include the following:

- It takes time to build a culture of interprofessional collaboration.

- It requires building relationships between and among team members.

- There are likely pockets of interprofessional collaborative practice that already exist within organizations. Highlight, resource, and spread them.

- Call out or name "interprofessional collaboration" so it is recognized as being different from how work may currently be done.

- Start small and build momentum.

- Create a culture by using multiple reinforcing practices.

Other successful strategies included putting patients first; demonstrating leadership commitment through words and actions; creating a level playing field, ensuring that all feel respected and valued; cultivating effective communication; hardwiring collaboration through organizational structure if possible; and investing in interprofessional education/continuing education.

A number of measurement tools are posted on the National Center for Interprofessional Practice and Collaboration (www.nexusipe.org) that can be used to assess current state or progress in evaluating culture. Tools may reflect evaluation of a specific practice setting such as the OR/surgery or may be more generalizable to different practice settings. Examples include Team Climate Inventory, Safety Organizing Scale, or the Interprofessional Socialization and Valuing Scale.

MOVING TOWARD AN INTEGRATED AND COLLABORATIVE ENVIRONMENT

Understanding that investing in and supporting IPCP can have a major impact on organizational excellence, how do we move from a system of hierarchy and silos to a system that is integrated and collaborative, with positive outcomes for nurses, teams, and patients? The

RWJF report describes how some high-performing organizations have started to change culture, but there must be a larger, more strategic effort to transform the healthcare system of today to one that meets the needs of the future. One strategy to advance IPCP acculturation is to redesign healthcare professions' education across the care continuum, from pre-licensure to postgraduate to continuing professional development. The following section provides a summary of recommendations for leaders in academia and in practice to implement changes in their respective organizations. Recommendations focus on transitioning siloed models of education to interprofessional models as a strategy to prepare and support a collaborative practice–ready healthcare workforce.

INTERPROFESSIONAL EDUCATION (IPE) AND INTERPROFESSIONAL CONTINUING EDUCATION (IPCE)

While interprofessional education (IPE) has been used to describe both academic and post-licensure education, the term interprofessional continuing education (IPCE) differentiates educational planning and evaluation that occurs in the pre-licensure academic curriculum (IPE) from that which occurs in the post-licensure practice-based continuum (IPCE).[10] IPE and IPCE share similar strategies as both require a planning process that reflects two or more professions working together, and both require opportunity for learners to learn from, with, and about each other. IPCE is distinct, however, in that it incorporates evaluation of practicing healthcare professionals, as well as outcomes that demonstrate the impact of an individual's performance on a team, performance of the team itself, or the impact of the team on patient and/or system results (www.jointaccreditation.org). In addition, the strategies used to design IPCE also address characteristics of the learning environment.

There is a long history of influential reports with calls to invest in team-based education as a strategy to improve collaboration in the practice setting. One of the first national reports was issued in 1972, and a brief overview of seminal documents highlights the increasing urgency expressed by thought leaders as well as national and international organizations.

The Institute of Medicine (IOM), now the National Academies of Sciences, Engineering, and Medicine (NAM), published a series of reports highlighting the need for education to improve collaborative practice. Starting with a report issued in 1972, *Educating for the Health Team: Report of the Conference on the Interrelationships of Educational Programs for Health Professions*, executive leaders from a variety of different professions described an education system that failed to prepare healthcare professionals for collaborative practice with a call to action to reform the education system and focus on team-based models.[11] The IOM continued to publish a series of seminal reports describing the current state of healthcare education and its impact on collaborative practice and patient outcomes.

In 1999, the IOM published *To Err is Human: Building a Safer Health System*, with recommendations to establish interdisciplinary team training programs, develop practice guidelines based on an interdisciplinary approach to care, and implement an interdisciplinary collaborative approach to redesigning complex systems of care.[12]

In 2001, *Crossing the Quality Chasm: A New Health System for the 21st Century* highlighted the need to coordinate care across teams of healthcare providers and between clinical settings.[13] Effective teams were described as communicating openly and collaboratively, having a sense of shared responsibility, and learning from their mistakes. The existing model of healthcare professional education was described as "siloed" by profession, resulting in providers being unprepared to practice in complex collaborative settings.

In 2003, *Health Professions Education: A Bridge to Quality* continued expanding on changes needed within the healthcare education continuum.[14] Healthcare professionals were not adequately prepared to practice collaboratively in teams, to implement quality improvement strategies, and to understand the complexities of system-wide practice. The report also called on accreditors, and licensing and certifying bodies to use their oversight processes as levers for change.

In 2010, the World Health Organization (WHO) published *Framework for Action on Interprofessional Education & Collaborative Practice,* the outcome of a WHO study group on interprofessional education and collaborative practice led by international experts in the field.[15] The report emphasized challenges that healthcare systems throughout the world were experiencing including fragmentation and unmet health needs. Interprofessional education was identified as a strategy to prepare a collaborative, practice-ready workforce (Figure 2.1). The report included a table of actions that individuals, leaders, hospitals, and systems could take to advance collaborative practice (Figure 2.2). The report also described mechanisms of action that shape interprofessional education and collaborative practice from the perspective of education, practice/environment, and health and education systems (Figure 2.3).

In 2010, *Redesigning Continuing Education in the Health Professions* was published by the IOM and focused specifically on the CPD system.[16] Recommendations included bringing health professionals from various disciplines together in carefully tailored learning environments and establishing a national center focused on interprofessional education.

In 2011, *The Future of Nursing: Leading Change, Advancing Health* was published with recommendations that nurses take leadership roles and work collaboratively with members from other professions in all practice settings across the healthcare continuum.[17]

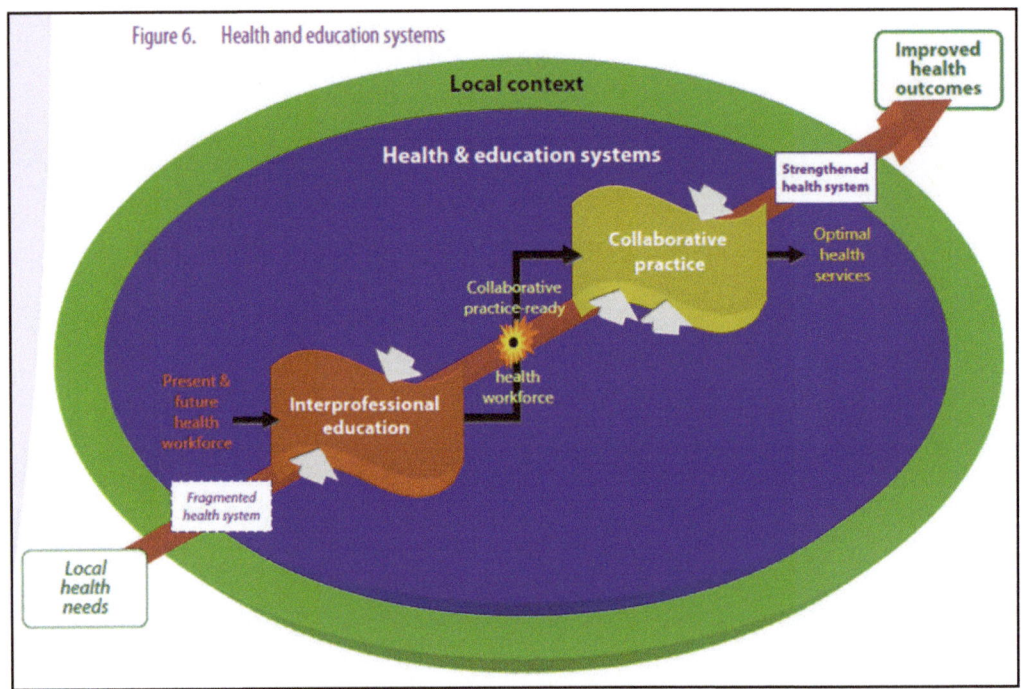

Figure 6. Health and education systems

Local context

Health & education systems

Improved
health
outcomes

Strengthened
health system

Collaborative
practice

Optimal
health
services

Collaborative
practice-ready

Present &
future
health
workforce

Interprofessional
education

health
workforce

Fragmented
health system

Local
health
needs

FIGURE 2.1

WHO, 2010 REPORT—INTERPROFESSIONAL EDUCATION AND COLLABORATIVE PRACTICE READY WORKFORCE

Reprinted from *Framework for action on interprofessional education & collaborative practice*, World Health Organization, Department of Human Resources for Health, "Learning together to work together for better health," Figure 6. Health and education systems, Page 18, Copyright 2010.

During this same period, the Interprofessional Education Collaborative (IPEC) was formed with representatives from medicine, nursing, pharmacy, dentistry, and public health. In 2010, IPEC released a set of core competencies in four domains that would form the basis for healthcare profession curricula in the future: Values/Ethics for Interprofessional Practice; Roles/Responsibilities; Interprofessional Communication; and Teams and Teamwork.[1]

In 2012, the National Center for Interprofessional Practice and Education was formed, a unique public-private partnership providing leadership, evidence, and resources needed to guide the nation on the use of interprofessional education and collaborative practice to enhance the experience of health care, improve population health, and reduce the overall cost of care. The National Center was founded by a grant from the Health Resources and Services Administration (HRSA) and is also supported in part by the Josiah Macy Jr. Foundation, the Robert Wood Johnson Foundation, the Gordon and Betty Moore Foundation, and the University of Minnesota (www.nexusipe.org). The National Center conducts a variety of activities designed to promote team-based education and practice and evaluate its impact on outcomes.

ACTION	PARTICIPANTS	LEVEL OF ENGAGEMENT EXAMPLES	POTENTIAL OUTCOMES
1. Structure processes that promote shared decision-making, regular communication, and community involvement	• Health facility managers and directors • Health workers	CONTEXTUALIZE • Discuss and share ideas for improved communication processes • Develop a sense of community through interaction and staff support	• A model of collaborative practice that recognizes the principles of shared decision-making and best practice in communication across professional boundaries
2. Design a built environment that promotes, foster, and extends interprofessional collaborative practice both withing and across service agencies	• Policy-makers • Health facility managers and directors • Health workers • Capital planners • Architects/space planners	CONTEXTUALIZE • Relocate and rearrange equipment to better facilitate communication flow	• Improved communication channels • Improved satisfaction among health workers
3. Develop personnel policies that recognize and support collaborative practice both within and across service agencies	• Government • Health facility managers and directors • Policy-makers • Regulatory/labor bodies	COMMIT • Review personnel policies and consider innovative remuneration and incentive plans	• Improved workplace health and well-being for workers • Improved working environment
4. Develop a delivery model that allows adequate time and space for staff to focus on interprofessional collaboration and delivery of care	• Health facility managers and directors • Policy-makers • Health workers	• Set aside time for staff to meet together to discuss cases, challenges, and successes • Provide opportunity for staff to be involved in development of new processes and strategic planning	• Improved interaction between management and staff • Greater cohesion and communications between health workers
5. Develop governance models that establish teamwork and shared responsibility for health-care service delivery between team members as the normative practice	• Health facility managers and directors • Policy-makers • Government leaders	CHAMPION • Review and update the existing governance model • Develop a strategic plan for an interprofessional education and collaborative practice model of care	• A sustained commitment to embedding interprofessional collaboration in the workplace • Updated governance model, job descriptions, vision, mission, and purpose

FIGURE 2.2
ACTIONS TO ADVANCE COLLABORATIVE PRACTICE

Reprinted from *Framework for action on interprofessional education & collaborative practice*, World Health Organization, Department of Human Resources for Health, "Moving forward," Table 1. Actions to advance interprofessional education for improved health outcomes, Page 27, Copyright 2010

INTERPROFESSIONAL EDUCATION	COLLABORATIVE PRACTICE	HEALTH AND EDUCATION SYSTEMS
Educator mechanisms • Champions • Institutional support • Managerial commitment • Shared objectives • Staff training **Curricular mechanisms** • Adult learning principles • Assessment • Compulsory attendance • Contextual learning • Learning outcomes • Logistics and scheduling • Programme content	**Institutional supports** • Governance models • Personnel policies • Shared operating procedures • Structured protocols • Supportive management practices **Working culture** • Communication strategies • Conflict resolution policies • Shared decision-making processes **Environment** • Built environment • Facilities • Space design	**Health-services delivery** • Capital planning • Commissioning • Financing • Funding streams • Remuneration models **Patient safety** • Accreditation • Professional registration • Regulation • Risk management

FIGURE 2.3
MECHANISMS TO SHAPE INTERPROFESSIONAL EDUCATION AND COLLABORATIVE PRACTICE

Reprinted from *Framework for action on interprofessional education & collaborative practice*, World Health Organization, Department of Human Resources for Health, "Moving forward," Table 4. Summary of identified mechanisms that shape interprofessional education and collaborative practice, Page 38, Copyright 2010

In 2013, a report from the Josiah Macy Jr. Foundation was published, *Transforming Patient Care: Aligning Interprofessional Education with Clinical Practice Redesign*.[18] Recommendations for immediate action included the following:

● Engage patients, families, and communities in the design, implementation, improvement, and evaluation of efforts to link interprofessional education and collaborative practice.

● Accelerate the design, implementation, and evaluation of innovative models linking interprofessional education and collaborative practice.

● Reform the education and lifelong career development of health professionals to incorporate interprofessional learning and team-based care.

● Revise professional regulatory standards and practices to permit and promote innovation in interprofessional education and collaborative practice.

● Realign existing resources to establish and sustain the linkage between interprofessional education and collaborative practice.

In 2015, the IOM published a study conducted by the Committee on Measuring the Impact of Interprofessional Education on Collaborative Practice and Patient Outcomes, Board on Global Health. The committee was charged with examining the impact of IPE on learners' knowledge, skills, and attitudes, and specifically to explore the relationship between IPE and performance in practice, including the impact on patient and population health and healthcare delivery system outcomes. The report, *Measuring the Impact of Interprofessional Education on Collaborative Practice and Patient Outcomes*, outlined four critical actions necessary for evaluating the impact of IPE on practice and outcomes. These included more closely aligning the education and healthcare delivery systems; developing a conceptual framework for measuring the impact of IPE; strengthening the evidence base for IPE; and linking IPE with changes in collaborative behavior. The committee also developed a conceptual model depicting the learning continuum from pre-licensure through CPD (Figure 2.4), and incorporated enabling or interfering factors as well as desired outcomes for individuals and health/health systems.[19]

In 2016, the National Academies published an update, *Assessing Progress on the Institute of Medicine Report The Future of Nursing*.[20] Recommendations included promoting nurses' interprofessional and lifelong learning and expanding efforts and opportunities for interprofessional collaboration and leadership development. The Joint Accreditation™ Program was

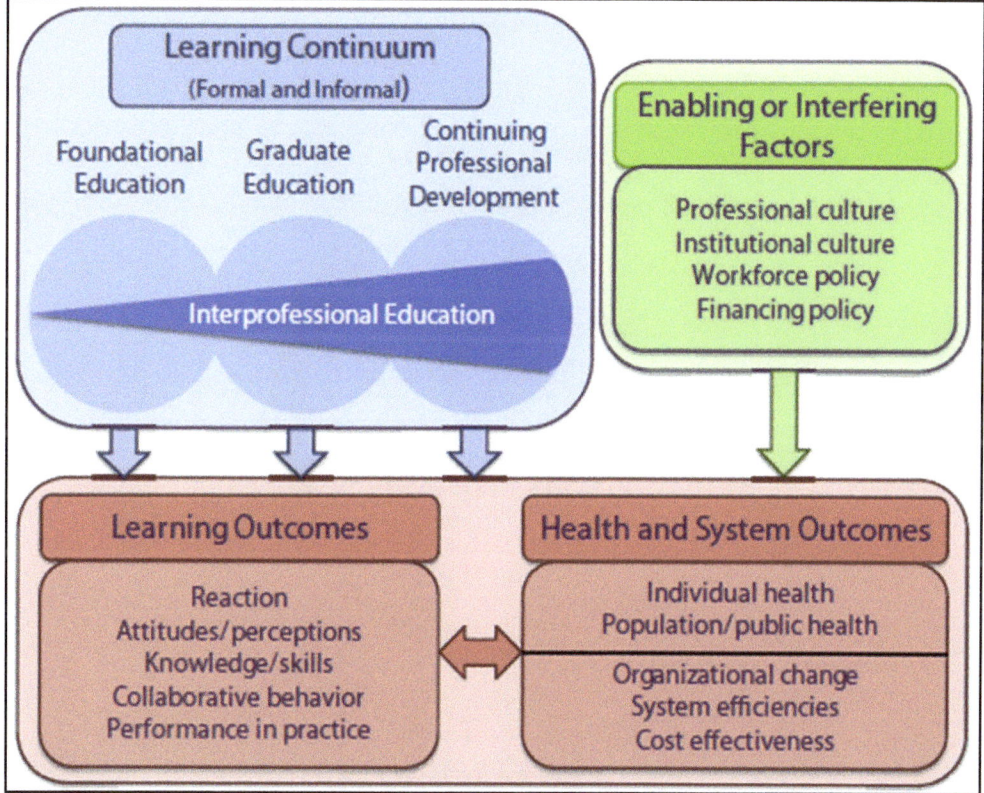

FIGURE 2.4
THE INTERPROFESSIONAL LEARNING CONTINUUM MODEL

Reprinted from: "Chapter 3, Conceptual Framework for Measuring the Impact of IPE" in *Measuring the Impact of Interprofessional Education on Collaborative Practice and Patient Outcomes* by Institute of Medicine, published 2015. Measuring the Impact of Interprofessional Education on Collaborative Practice and Patient Outcomes.

specifically cited in the report as a strategy for increasing nurses' access and participation in IPCE. The report also included recommendations that the Center for Medicare & Medicaid Innovation (CMMI) supports for developing models of care that use nurses in a leadership capacity, and for healthcare organizations and nursing leaders to support nurses in developing and adopting innovative, patient-centered care models. The American Association of Medical Colleges (AAMC) was commended for creating its MedEdPORTAL® and expanding it to incorporate interprofessional learning resources and educational materials (https://www.mededportal.org/).

In 2016, the IPEC competencies were also updated, newly organized around a singular domain of Interprofessional Collaboration and explicitly linking to the Triple Aim[6] (Figure 2.5). The competency domains are reflected in the Table 2.1.[2]

In 2018, the Josiah Macy Jr. Foundation explored how characteristics of a high-quality learning environment support optimal learning and better alignment with patient needs and societal goals for better health in the report *Improving Environments for Learning in the Health Professions*.[21] One recommendation from the report called on health professions education and healthcare organizations, the federal government, and foundations to collaborate to

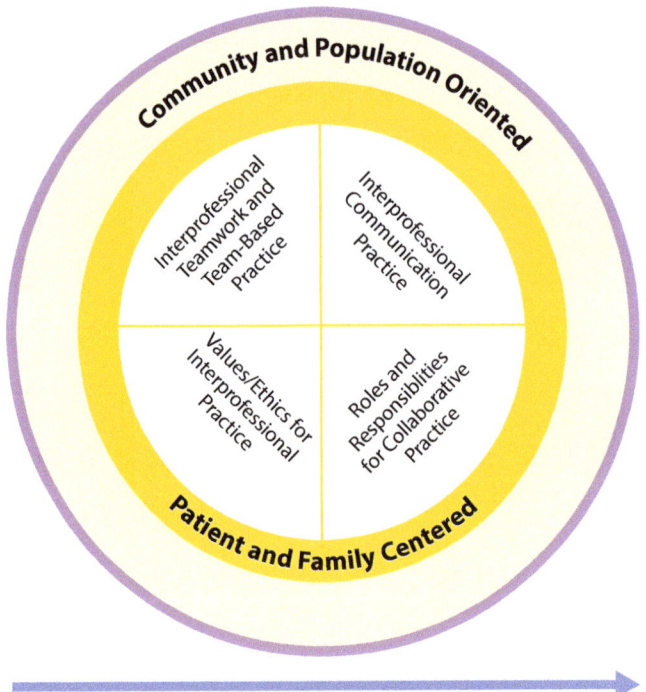

The Learning Continuum—pre-licensure through practice trajectory

FIGURE 2.5
INTERPROFESSIONAL COLLABORATION COMPETENCY DOMAIN

Reprinted from Interprofessional Education Collaborative. (2016). Core Competencies for Interprofessional Collaborative Practice: 2016 Update. Washington, DC. Interprofessional Education Collaborative.

TABLE 2.1
COMPETENCY DOMAINS

Competency 1
Work with individuals of other professions to maintain a climate of mutual respect and shared values. (Values/Ethics for Interprofessional Practice)
Competency 2
Use the knowledge of one's own role and those of other professions to appropriately assess and address the health care needs of patients and to promote and advance the health of populations. (Roles/Responsibilities)
Competency 3
Communicate with patients, families, communities, and professionals in health and other fields in a responsive and responsible manner that supports a team approach to the promotion and maintenance of health and the prevention and treatment of disease. (Interprofessional Communication)
Competency 4
Apply relationship-building values and the principles of team dynamics to perform effectively in different team roles to plan, deliver, and evaluate patient/population-centered care and population health programs and policies that are safe, timely, efficient, effective, and equitable. (Teams and Teamwork)

advance the nation's learning environments. The National Collaborative for Improving the Clinical Learning Environment (NCICLE) was cited as an example of a recently organized collaborative. NCICLE reports, available at www.ncicle.org, highlight the need to prepare learners to engage in safe and effective interprofessional collaborative care[21] (Figure 2.6).

In summary, transforming organizations to achieve excellence will require collaboration across professions. IPE and IPCE are strategies to achieve that goal. From early entry into pre-licensure programs and over a career of practice, nurses and other healthcare professionals must learn together to practice together.

Burnout

One driver behind the increased focus on IPCP is the high prevalence of burnout and depression among healthcare students and practitioners across all professions. Studies report the incidence of burnout/emotional exhaustion in nurses to be as high as 43% and twice the rate of depression as compared to other US workers.[22] Burnout has been associated with an increased rate of medical errors, healthcare-associated infections, and patient deaths. Job dissatisfaction, intent to leave, and loss of productivity worsen with burnout. Alcohol/substance abuse, suicidal ideation, and suicide increase with burnout. The National Academies of Medicine created a resource center to share knowledge to combat poor clinician well-being (https://nam.edu/clinicianwellbeing/resource-center/). Resources reflecting the positive impact of team-based care and collaboration on reducing burnout and improving outcomes can be found on the site. The site also includes measurement tools that can be used to evaluate burnout or well-being such as the Copenhagen Burnout Inventory, the Well-Being Index Self-Assessment Tool, or the Work-Life Balance Quiz.

Components of Learning Environments	ELEMENTS TO BE CONSIDERED
Personal	• Who are the individuals ("learners," e.g., trainees, teachers, supervisors, staff, patients, etc.) in the LE being studied? • How are LEs described, taking into consideration elements of diversity and equity (e.g., personal histories, race/ethnicity, disability, gender identity, academic and/or work backgrounds)? • How would the individuals describe themselves? • How will individual learning, or performance, be assessed? • What are learners' perceptions of the LE?
Social	• What types of interpersonal interactions, including collaborations and conflicts, occur in the LE (consider patients, as well as intraprofessional, interprofessional, and staff members in the LE)? • What are the instructional strategies and pedagogical approaches used in the LE (consider formal, informal, and hidden elements)?
Organizational	• What organizational structures, practices, language, rituals, policies, norms, and routines are being investigated? • How aligned are the educational and clinical missions and practices? • What are the organizational resources, structures, and leadership? • What populations are served (patients, learners)?
Physical and Virtual Spaces	• What are the locations and qualities of the LE being studied (classroom, virtual, simulation, clinical workplace)? • What characteristics of the physical/virtual space influence learning? • What is the role of technology in the LE?

FIGURE 2.6
ELEMENTS TO CONSIDER IN DESIGNING STUDIES OF LEARNING ENVIRONMENTS

Reprinted from Irby, D.M. Improving Environments for Learning in the Health Professions. Proceedings of a conference sponsored by Josiah Macy Jr. Foundation in April 2018; New York, NY: Josiah Macy Jr. Foundation, 2018.

TOOLS, RESOURCES, AND STRATEGIES TO PROMOTE IPCP

Based on an abundance of evidence that promoting IPCP can have a positive impact on the health and well-being of nurses, teams, and patients, how can nursing leaders successfully transform individuals, units, organizations, and systems from single-profession and siloed models to interprofessional team-based models of care? What frameworks currently exist and how can they be operationalized across different healthcare settings and continuously rotating teams?

Individuals

Teams are a collection of individuals who each possess their own characteristics, skills, and weaknesses. Teams form and re-form continuously in the healthcare system, presenting unique challenges for nursing leaders. One first step that nursing leaders can employ to impact IPCP is building the skill sets of individual team members. From frontline staff to executive leaders, and across professions, investing in team-based education provides an opportunity for individuals to learn from, with, and about each other.

In the practice setting, individuals should have the opportunity to regularly participate in IPCE. While some problems in practice are best addressed through single-profession models of education, the vast majority of issues in the healthcare setting impact and require the contribution of multiple professionals to effectively effect change. A conceptual framework proposed by Moore and colleagues provides an overview and guiding principles that can be applied to single profession as well as interprofessional continuing education. Outcomes are assessed at levels that include learning, competence, transfer, performance, patient health, and population health[23] (Figure 2.7).

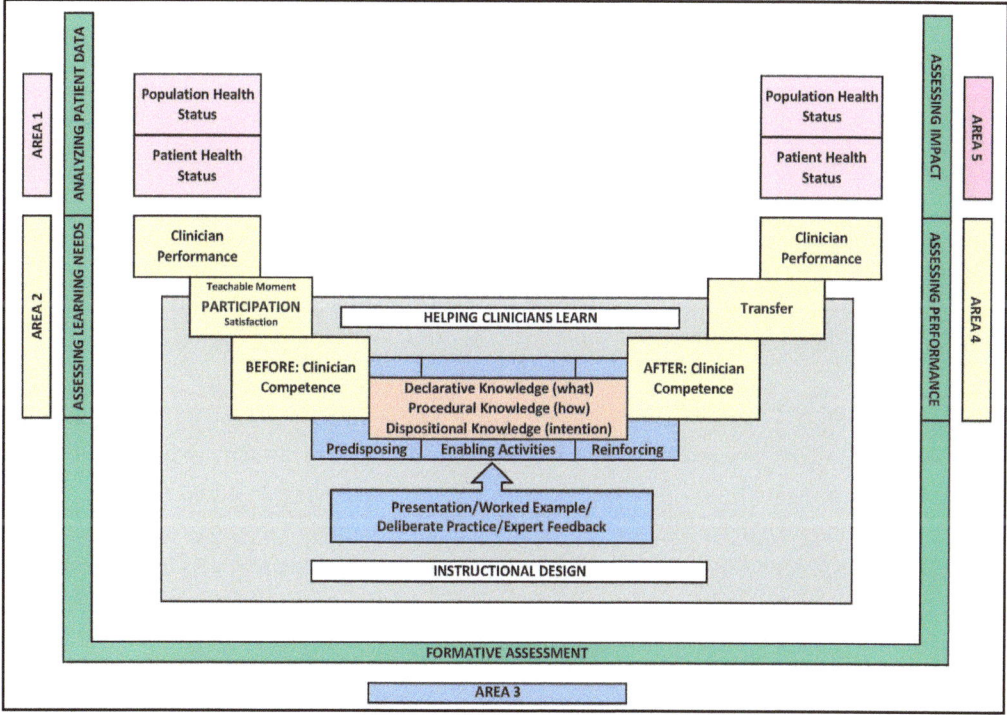

FIGURE 2.7
CONCEPTUAL FRAMEWORK FOR PLANNING LEARNING ACTIVITIES AND ASSESSING LEARNERS IN IPCE

Reprinted from Moore, D. E., Chappell, K. B., Sherman, L., & Vinayaga-Pavan, M. (2018). A conceptual framework for planning and assessing learning in continuing education activities designed for clinicians in one profession and/or clinical teams. *Medical Teacher, 40*(9), 904–913.

In addition to the framework, Weaver and colleagues [24] outlined considerations for IPCE that are critical for success for adult learners:

- Emphasize the value proposition

- Approach from a systems perspective

- Develop faculty/educator skills

- Incorporate active learning strategies

- Create a safe environment

- Use practical, meaningful scenarios

- Build time for practice and reflection

- Incorporate team skills in practical ways

- Use formative and summative evaluation

- Reinforce skills used in daily practice

Implementing reminders into activity-planning documents helps reinforce the critical elements that distinguish IPCE from single-profession education.

Organizations

Within organizations and systems, how can nursing leaders create a culture that supports IPCP? What strategies "hard wire" collaborative practice models? Several tools exist to help nursing leaders evaluate practice settings and implement strategies to promote collaborative practice. The Interprofessional Collaborative Organizational Map and Preparedness Assessment (IP-COMPASS) is one such resource.[25] IP-COMPASS is a quality improvement framework that helps healthcare organizations create an environment that supports IPE/IPCE and IPCP. It is designed to increase understanding of the organizational culture that can create an environment that is conducive to interprofessional learning. The National Center for Interprofessional Practice and Education's Resource Center includes a toolkit specifically designed for preceptors in the practice setting to learn how to effectively provide interprofessional learning experiences. The toolkit can be found at https://nexusipe.org/informing/about-national-center/news/toolkit-prepares-preceptors-interprofessional-teams-learners. The Resource Center also includes a variety of archived webinars that can be accessed at no charge.

ROLE OF CREDENTIALING ORGANIZATIONS IN PROMOTING IPCP

The ANCC credentialing programs value, promote, and require nursing leaders to embrace IPCP. Using credentialing as a driver for change, ANCC has implemented expectations for IPCP at the individual, program, and organization levels.

ANCC Accreditation Program

The ANCC Accreditation Program's four distinct credentials provide a foundation for collaborative practice. Two credentials distinctly recognize IPCE and IPCP in standards, the Joint Accreditation™ Program administered collaboratively with accreditor colleagues in medicine and pharmacy, and the Practice Transition Accreditation™ Program.

Joint Accreditation™

Joint Accreditation™ for Interprofessional Continuing Education offers organizations the opportunity to be simultaneously accredited to provide medical, nursing, optometry, pharmacy, physician assistants, psychology, and social work continuing education through a single, unified application process, fee structure, and set of accreditation standards. The program continues to add professions. The goal of the program is to promote IPCE specifically designed to improve IPCP in healthcare delivery. In 2019, almost 100 organizations have achieved this innovative and unique credential, including two organizations outside the United States. The program leaders have produced a series of leadership summit reports, funded in part by the Josiah Macy Jr. Foundation, that describe how this community of practice is advancing its mission. The three reports are available on the program web site at www.jointaccreditation.org:

- *IPCE Works! Identifying Measures of Success and Evaluating Our Impact*—Report from the 2018 Joint Accreditation™ Leadership Summit

- *Promoting Research Across the Continuum of Health Professions Education: Making Patient Care Better*—Report from the 2017 Joint Accreditation™ Leadership Summit

- *By the Team for the Team: Evolving Interprofessional Continuing Education™ for Optimal Patient Care*—Report from the 2016 Joint Accreditation™ Leadership Summit

Key recommendations from each report are outlined for the reader, and reports include numerous case studies and examples submitted by jointly accredited providers.

The 2016 report key recommendations focused on creating and sustaining a successful IPCE program. They included developing buy-in from leadership; ensuring that an IPCE program aligned with and supported the organization's mission; building an IPCE team and modeling best practices for others; incorporating patients as members of the healthcare team; implementing a phased-in approach to transition from single-profession to inter-professional education; focusing on high-quality strategic team interventions; measuring outcomes of IPCE activities; and communicating the value of IPCE widely.

Recommendations from the 2017 report reflected a focus on increasing the rigor of evaluation methodologies, moving from anecdotes to thoughtfully designed studies with demonstrated outcomes. Creating an evaluation or research plan including funding strategies, developing organizational partnerships, and disseminating results were identified by jointly accredited providers as critical for success.

The 2018 report, widely requested by jointly accredited providers, focused on evaluation. Key lessons included identifying the specific team performance areas that need improvement; using resources such as those provided by the National Center to design evaluation; linking educational content to skills and strategies needed for team practice; revising evaluation strategies to reflect the team rather than the individual; giving patients a key role in designing IPCE; considering strategies for evaluation that are less burdensome for the learner; and partnering with organizations to collect practice level and patient outcome data.

Collectively, the reports demonstrate how organizations that have pursued Joint Accreditation™ have positively impacted practice and patient outcomes, supporting the Future of Nursing recommendations.

Practice Transition Accreditation™ Program

ANCC's Practice Transition Accreditation™ Program sets standards for RN and APRN residency and fellowship programs. Criteria require program directors to embed content on collaboration into curricula and to support residents and fellows in developing individual and team-based skills.

For nurses, the transition to practice has long been recognized as an intensely stressful period. Marlene Kramer first described the challenges new graduate nurses face in her book *Reality Shock.*[26] Today, newly graduated nurses enter practice environments that are extremely demanding and require a high degree of clinical proficiency, critical thinking ability, and clinical leadership skill. Nurse residency and fellowship programs help mitigate the stress of transition by incorporating activities that improve clinical skills, critical thinking and clinical reasoning skills, time management, and delegation skills. These programs also help reduce high levels of turnover and vacancy within organizations, as well as the loss of RNs within the profession.[27-28] Accrediting bodies for nurse residency and fellowship programs have embedded criteria that directly address identified stressors through, for example, programs to help the trainees manage stress and role transition. Residents and fellows learn to manage time, improve communication skills, and work as members of the interprofessional care team while developing strategies to prevent compassion fatigue, promote resiliency, and address ethical dilemmas.

Accredited PTAP programs demonstrate interprofessional collaboration through quality improvement projects or evidence-based-practice projects, simulation experiences, or active participation in interprofessional rounds. Many programs create experiences where team members can get to know each other through storytelling or learning about each other's roles as a member of the team. Collaboration and teamwork in transition-to-practice programs enable nurses to practice, learn, and improve upon their skills in order to improve the clinical environment and patient outcomes.

ANCC Pathway to Excellence™ Program and Pathway to Excellence Long Term Care®

ANCC's Pathway to Excellence™ Program recognizes organizations that have demonstrated a positive practice environment for nurses and for the other members of the healthcare team. Program standards and elements of performance emphasize the importance of nursing leadership and nurses' contributions to establishing and maintaining a culture of interprofessional collaboration and collaborative practice.

- **Standard 1**. "Organizations achieving Pathway to Excellence® designation have an established shared governance structure as the foundation for involving direct care nurses in decision-making. Allowing direct care nurse input into decision-making influences care delivery, work flow, hiring, and product evaluation. Interprofessional collaboration is also integral within the organization, engaging staff, building teamwork, and strengthening the shared governance culture."[30]

- **Element of Performance (EOP) 3.1**: "Describe how interprofessional decision-making is utilized in the process to transition patients from one level of care to another; and provide one example of how the interprofessional collaboration process impacted a patient care transition."[30]

Nurses from Pathway organizations have described improvement in communication, team-work, and coordination of care across the continuum resulting in better patient outcomes, enhanced patient experience, collegial relationships among the different disciplines, and increased employee satisfaction.

ANCC Magnet Recognition™ Program

ANCC's Magnet Recognition™ Program, an outcomes-based credential awarded to health-care organizations that demonstrate nursing excellence and quality patient care, incorpo-rates standards and sources of evidence with empirical outcomes that reflect a commit-ment to IPCE and IPCP. Nursing leaders in Magnet organizations are expected to be equal and collaborative partners within the executive leadership team and to ensure that nurses at all levels are engaged in interprofessional decision-making groups.

- **Standard**: "Exemplary professional practice in Magnet-recognized organizations is evidenced by effective and efficient care services, interprofessional collaboration, and high-quality patient outcomes. Magnet nurses' partner with patients, families, support systems, and interprofessional teams to positively impact patient care and outcomes. Interprofessional team members include but are not limited to personnel from medicine, pharmacy, nutrition, rehabilitation, social work, psychology, and other professions that collaborate to ensure a comprehensive plan of care."[31]

- **Source of Evidence (EP5)**: "Provide one example with supporting evidence, of nurses participation in interprofessional collaborative practice to ensure coordination of care across the spectrum of healthcare services." [31]

- **Source of Evidence (EP6EO)**: "Provide one example, with supporting evidence, of an improvement in a defined patient population outcome associated with nurse participa-tion in an interprofessional collaborative plan of care." [31]

ANCC Certification Program

And finally, ANCC's board certification exams for RNs and APRNs across multiple specialty practice areas reflect expectations that all nurses promote and participate in IPCP (https://www.nursingworld.org/certification/).

ANCC also launched its first interprofessional board certification exam—a competency-based interprofessional entry-level examination, National Healthcare Disaster Certification.

A competency-based interprofessional examination, it provides a valid and reliable assessment of the knowledge, skills, and competencies of healthcare professionals relevant to all phases of the disaster preparedness, mitigation, response, and recovery cycles. The goal of this exam is to promote successful outcomes for the public, disaster responders, and healthcare professionals involved in a disaster.

Examples of how IPCP is integrated into the Test Content Outline (TCO) domains of ANCC's exams reflect how items are included to evaluate knowledge and skills in the area of interprofessional collaborative practice.

- Leadership (APRN specialty exam)
  - Knowledge of:
    - Principles and concepts of interprofessional and intradisciplinary practice
  - Skills in:
    - Fostering collaboration with multiple stakeholders to improve health care
    - Building and leading collaborative interprofessional care teams

- Health Promotion (RN specialty exam)
  - Skills in:
    - Identifying and prioritizing of learning needs (e.g., health literacy, patient expectations, family-centered care)
    - Developing a collaborative education plan with the individual, family, significant other, caregiver, and interdisciplinary team

SUMMARY

Over the past decade, there has been substantial progress in aligning the education–practice continuum and promoting IPCP. Accreditation standards for academic programs and postgraduate residency and fellowship programs require organizations to include IPE and IPCE activities for learners. In the practice setting, the Joint Accreditation™ Program incentivizes organizations to develop IPCE activities, and the number of applicants and professions that have embraced this innovative accreditation attest to its success. Single professional accreditors in CPD have embedded IPCE into standards for commendation, incentivizing educational providers with stretch goals. Collaboration among associations and accreditors across professions is historic. There remain barriers to widespread adoption, however, that will need to be addressed to fully embrace new models of education and care delivery.

Financial models within academia and practice can be perceived as barriers to interprofessional education and collaboration. When students from multiple professions are integrated into a single educational model, who "owns" the revenue from tuition? When professions are paid on a fee-for-service model and have few incentives to engage in IPCE, how do you get them to embrace participating? Issues such as these will have to be resolved to successfully move forward.

As the healthcare system evolves from a fee-for-service model to one that is rewarded based on outcomes, there is more incentive for organizations to implement strategies to improve interprofessional collaboration. The evidence base that supports the relationship between IPE/IPCP, IPCP, practice change, and positive patient outcomes continues to grow. Successful organizations must embrace IPCP to achieve excellence.

ANCC's organizational credentials provide a framework to support IPCP. Educational providers that achieve Joint Accreditation™ or Accreditation with Distinction in continuing nursing education have demonstrated the ability to provide high quality IPCE. Hospitals and healthcare systems that achieve the Pathway to Excellence® and Magnet Recognition® credentials have integrated interprofessional collaboration into the organization and have examples that demonstrate their success.

Nursing leaders are well positioned to use these resources and others to achieve organizational excellence. They can transform the healthcare system of today to one that meets the needs of the future.

DEFINITIONS

Interprofessional Education: "When students from two or more professions learn about, from and with each other to enable effective collaboration and improve health outcomes."[15]

Interprofessional Collaborative Practice: "When multiple health workers from different professional backgrounds work together with patients, families, carers [sic], and communities to deliver the highest quality of care."[15]

Interprofessional Continuing Education: "When members from two or more professions learn about, from and with each other to enable effective collaboration and improve health outcomes." (www.jointaccreditation.org)

REFERENCES

1. Interprofessional Education Collaborative Expert Panel. (2011). Core competencies for interprofessional collaborative practice: Report of an expert panel. Washington, D.C.: Interprofessional Education Collaborative.

2. Interprofessional Education Collaborative. (2016). Core competencies for interprofessional collaborative practice: 2016 update. Washington, DC: Interprofessional Education Collaborative.

3. Chappell, K., Holmboe, E., and Remondet-Wall, J. (2018). The role of health care professions' accreditors in promoting well-being across the learning continuum. NAM Perspectives. Discussion Paper. National Academy of Medicine, Washington, DC. https://nam.edu/the-role-of-health-care-professions'-accreditors-in-promoting-well-being-across -the-learning-continuum (in press).

4. Chappell, K., Regnier, K., & Travlos, D. (2018). Leading by example: The role of accreditors in promoting interprofessional collaborative practice, *Journal of Interprofessional Care*, DOI: 10.1080/13561820.2018.1433276

5. Bodenheimer, Thomas & Sinsky, Christine. (2014). From Triple to Quadruple Aim: Care of the Patient Requires Care of the Provider. *Annals of Family Medicine*. 12. 573–576. 10.1370/afm.1713.

6. Berwick, D.M., Nolan, T.WI, & Whittington, J. (2008). The triple aim: Care, health and cost. *Health Affairs*, 27(3), 759–769.

7. Barr, Koppel, Reeves, Hammick and Freeth (2005) *Effective Interprofessional Education: Argument, Assumption and Evidence*. Blackwell Publishing and CAIPE

8. Reeves, S., S. Fletcher, H. Barr, I. Birch, S. Boet, N. Davies, A. McFadyen, J. Rivera, and S. C. Kitto. 2016. A BEME systematic review of the effects of interprofessional education: BEME Guide No. 39. *Medical Teacher* 38(7):656–668.

9. Fauteux, N. & Ladden, M.D. (2015). *The value of nursing in building a culture of health* (Part 1). Robert Wood Johnson Foundation.

10. Harper, M. & Maloney, P. (Eds). (2016). *Nursing professional development: Scope and standards of practice* (3rd ed.). Chicago, IL: Association for Nursing Professional Development.

11. Institute of Medicine. (1972). *Educating for the Health Team. Report of the Conference on the Interrelationships of Educational Programs for Health Professionals*. Washington, DC: National Academy of Sciences. October 2–3.

12. Kohn, L.T., Corrigan, J.M., & Donaldson, M.S. (Eds). (1999). *To Err is Human: Building a Safer Health System*. Washington, DC: National Academy Press.

13. Institute of Medicine: Committee on Quality of Healthcare in America, Institute of Medicine (2001). *Crossing the Quality Chasm: A New Health System for the 21st Century*. Washington, DC: National Academy Press.

14. Greiner, A.C., & Knebel, E. (Eds). (2003). *Health Professions Education: A Bridge to Quality*. Washington DC: National Academy Press.

15. World Health Organization. (2010). *Framework for Action on Interprofessional Education & Collaborative Practice*. WHO Press. Accessed at: http://whqlibdoc.who.int/hq/2010/WHO_HRH_HPN_10.3_eng.pdf?ua=1

16. Institute of Medicine. (2010). *Redesigning Continuing Education in the Health Professions.* Washington, DC: The National Academies Press.

17. Institute of Medicine. (2011). *The future of nursing: Leading change, advancing health.* Institute of Medicine and Robert Wood Johnson Foundation.

18. Josiah Macy Jr. Foundation, Transforming Patient Care, 2013

19. Institute of Medicine. 2015. Measuring the Impact of Interprofessional Education on Collaborative Practice and Patient Outcomes. https://doi.org/10.17226/21726. Reprinted with permission from the National Academy of Sciences, Courtesy of the National Academies Press, Washington, D.C.

20. National Academies of Sciences, Engineering, and Medicine. 2016. *Assessing Progress on the Institute of Medicine Report: The Future of Nursing.* Washington, DC: The National Academies Press.

21. Irby, D.M. Improving Environments for Learning in the Health Professions. Proceedings of a conference sponsored by Josiah Macy Jr. Foundation in April 2018; New York, NY: Josiah Macy Jr. Foundation, 2018.

22. Dyrbye, L.N., Shanafelt, T.D., Sinsky, C.A., Cipriano, P.F., Bhatt, J., Ommaya, A., West, C.P., & Meyers, D. (July 5, 2017). Burnout among health care professionals: A call to explore and address this underrecognized threat to safe, high-quality care. Discussion Paper. National Academy of Medicine.

23. Moore, D.E., Chappell, K.B., Sherman, L., & Vinayaga-Pavan, M. (2018). A conceptual framework for planning and assessing learning in continuing education activities designed for clinicians in one profession and/or clinical teams. *Medical Teacher* online accessed at: https://www.tandfonline.com/doi/full/10.1080/0142159X.2018.1483578

24. Weaver, S.J., Rosen, M.A., Salas, E., Baum, K.D., & King, H.B. (2010). Integrating the Science of Team Training: Guidelines for Continuing Education. *Journal of Continuing Education in the Health Professions*, 30(4), 208–220.

25. Parker, K., Jacobson, A., McGuire, M., Zorzi, R., and Oandasan, I. (2012). How to build high-quality interprofessional education in your hospital: the IP-COMPASS tool. *Quality Management Health Care*, 21(3), 160–168.

26. Kramer, M. 1974. *Reality shock: Why nurses leave nursing.* St. Louis, MO: C. V. Mosby.

27. Ulrich B., C. Krozek, S. Early, C. H. Ashlock, L. M. Africa, M. L. Carman. 2010. Improving Retention, Confidence, And Competence of New Graduate Nurses: Results from a 10-Year Longitudinal Database. *Nursing Economics* 28(6):336–375

28. Goode C. J., K. S. Glassman, P.R. Ponte, M. Krugman, T. Peterman. 2018. Requiring a nurse residency for newly licensed registered nurses. *Nursing Outlook* 66(3):329–332.

29. Chappell, K.B. (2016). The Clinical Learning Environment: Improving the Education Experience and Patient Outcomes Within Magnet® Organizations. *JONA*, 46(1), 1– 3.

30. American Nurses Credentialing Center. (2019). *2016 Pathway to Excellence Application Manual.* Silver Spring, MD.:Author.

31. American Nurses Credentialing Center. (2019). *2019 Magnet Application Manual.* Silver Spring, MD.:Author.

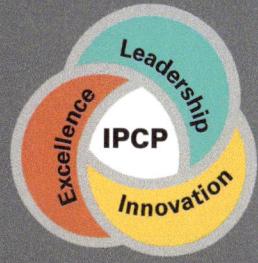

BUILDING A FRAMEWORK FOR SUCCESS

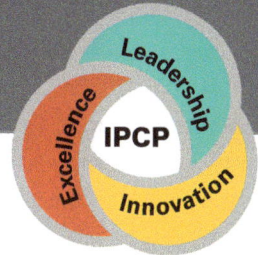

BUILDING A FRAMWORK FOR SUCCESS

Authentic leaders are not made nor are they born; they are enabled or disabled by the organizations in which they work.

—David Leach, MD (Past Executive Director, ACGME)

USING IPCP AND PROFESSIONAL PRACTICE MODELS TO DRIVE ORGANIZATIONAL EXCELLENCE

Step 2 presents core components of a robust IPCP model. As organizations consider how to implement collaborative practices, it is necessary to consider how the nursing profession organizes teams. The nursing profession utilizes a professional practice model (PPM) framework to create an environment of nursing excellence. Many people misunderstand what a PPM is and how it can be operationalized within an organization and within IPCP teams. There are two main sections to this step. The first focuses on the who, what, why, and how of developing a PPM. The second discusses strategies in developing, disseminating, and enculturating the model into the nursing strategic plan and into practice.

RECOMMENDED READING

Cobb, S., Wolf, K., Shine, C., Jadwin, A. (2018). Involving clinical nurses in evaluation of a professional practice model: A focus group research study approach. *Journal of Nursing Administration*, 48(9), 466–468.

DEFINING PROFESSIONAL PRACTICE MODELS (PPM)

The American Nurses Credentialing Center's (ANCC's) *Magnet ® Manual* defines a PPM as **"the driving force of nursing care. It is a schematic description of a system, theory, or phenomenon that depicts how nurses practice, collaborate, communicate, and develop professionally to provide the highest-quality care for those served by the organization (e.g., patients, families, communities)."**[1] (p. 158). The literature describes professional practice models as a way to visualize how a nursing division operates.[2] Hoffart and Woods define a PPM as "a system (structure, process, and values) that supports registered nurse control over the delivery of nursing care and the environment in which care is delivered"[3] (p. 354). The American Nurses Association's (ANA's) *Nursing Professional Development: Scope and Standards of Practice* helps guide organizations when trying to further define PPM components. For those organizations on the Journey to Magnet Excellence®, the *Magnet Manual* focuses on two specific standards* (EP1EO and EP2EO) in relation to the involvement of clinical nurses and the PPM. Applicants achieving standards EP1EO and EP2EO must describe and demonstrate clinical nurse involvement in development, implementation, and evaluation of the PPM. Standard EP1EO requires examples of clinical nurses providing evidence-based change. Standard EP2EO evaluates the impact of the PPM on the nursing division through nursing satisfaction data. Exhibit 3.1 provides an overview of PPM dimensions.

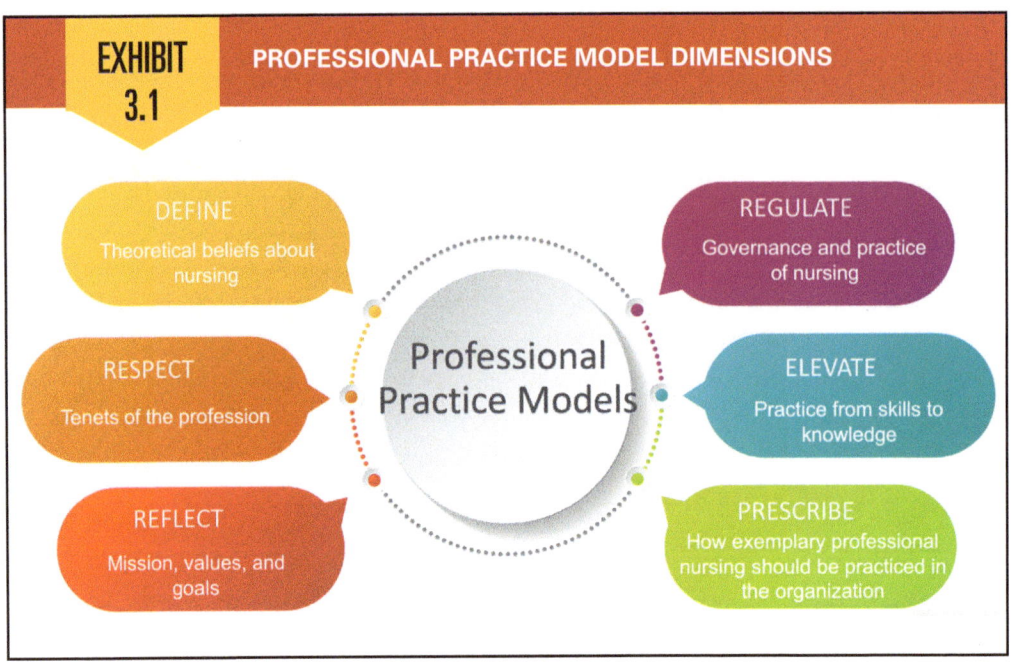

EXHIBIT 3.1 — **PROFESSIONAL PRACTICE MODEL DIMENSIONS**

DEFINE
Theoretical beliefs about nursing

REGULATE
Governance and practice of nursing

RESPECT
Tenets of the profession

ELEVATE
Practice from skills to knowledge

REFLECT
Mission, values, and goals

PRESCRIBE
How exemplary professional nursing should be practiced in the organization

Professional Practice Models

---

* These standards are based on the 2019 Magnet ® Application Manual. For Magnet Recognition Program® updates and developments, please refer to https://www.nursingworld.org/organizational-programs/magnet/

BASIC COMPONENTS OF A PPM

All PPMs should incorporate components that are fundamental to organizational success. For example, Hoffart and Woods state that the PPM should have components focused on professional relationships, the patient care delivery system, management approach, and compensation and rewards.[3] Wolf, Aukerman, and Boland describe PPM components as having transformational leadership, care delivery systems, professional growth, and collaborative practice in their Transformational Model for Professional Practice.[4] Making a PPM meet the needs of the organization is also important. For example, some organizations have included evidence-based practice and research as an individual core component because of the increased focus of new knowledge and innovation in the *Magnet Manual*. However, a review of many PPMs reveals seven core components that appear in almost all (Exhibit 3.2). These components are the following:

- Mission
- Vision
- Values
- How an organization manages and governs
- How an organization cares for its patients
- How various professions relate to each other
- How an organization develops and recognizes employees

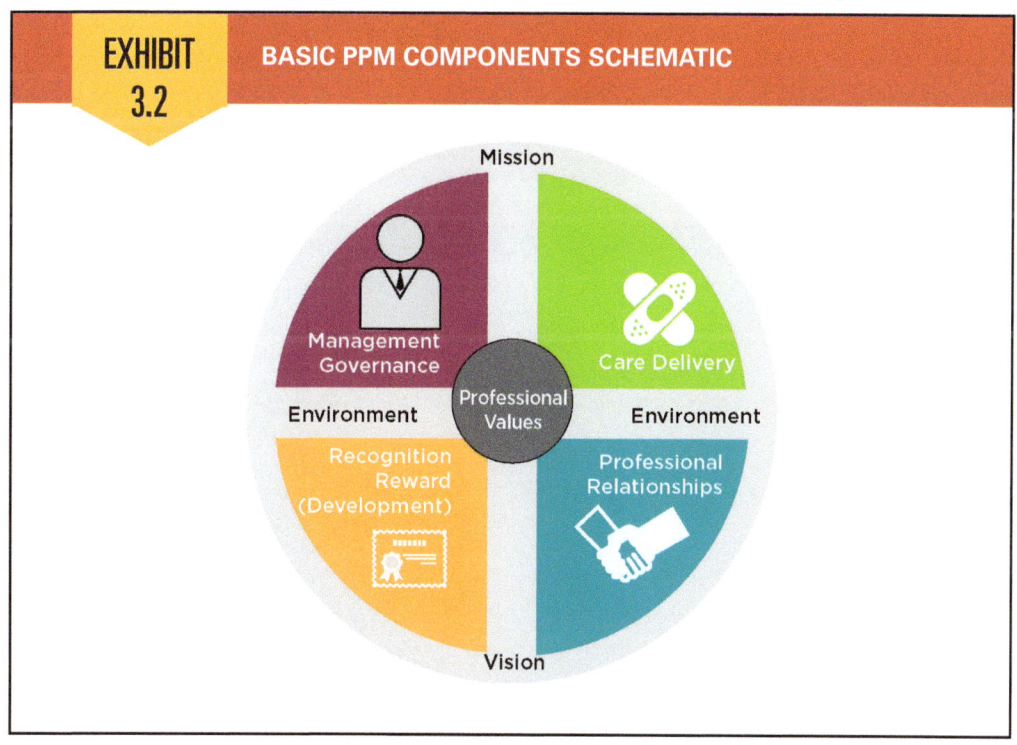

EXHIBIT 3.2 **BASIC PPM COMPONENTS SCHEMATIC**

DEFINING THE CORE ELEMENTS

An organization's mission, vision, and values set the direction of the entire organization. It is essential that nursing's mission and vision are aligned with the organization's. Otherwise, employees will become confused as to what the key priorities are and where they are headed in the future.

> **Mission**: A brief description of an organization's fundamental purpose. Why does the organization exist?

> **Vision**: A picture of the organization in the future. Where is the organization going?

> **Values**: Shared beliefs or ideals about what is good and desirable in practice as well as what is not. Personal values drive one's behavior. Group values drive practice.

Examples of values may include words such as excellence, caring, trust, honesty, efficiency, collegiality, patient safety, and creativity. Leaders and staff need to test their values. Employees have trouble buying into values that aren't really practiced. If the organization values transparency, for example, employees would expect to see near misses as learning opportunities. If an organization values staff engagement, staff should have time and support to attend shared governance meetings and other committees where their voices are heard. An organization valuing community involvement would want to make sure employees are involved and supported in community initiatives.

An easy way to choose values is through the use of the nominal technique. The nominal technique, shown in Exercise 3.1, gives participants an opportunity to contribute to developing unit-, division-, or organization-level values. If used correctly, the exercise will make participants feel that an important part of their personal value system is now vested in the organization.

EXERCISE 3.1 — NOMINAL GROUP TECHNIQUE WHEN CREATING VALUES

1. Give all group members five sticky notes on which to write their five top values.
2. Have each person place their notes on a wall.
3. Categorize identical responses and then write each value on its own large sticky note.
4. Give all group members three dot stickers and ask them to place their dots on the values they feel are most important to have within the nursing division.
5. Keep narrowing down the values until you reach consensus.

LEADERSHIP AND GOVERNANCE

Staff need to know how an organization makes decisions and the structures and processes through which nursing's voice is heard to know how their input impacts patient outcomes. Several models of leadership exist; however, in the past 15 years, more and more organizations understand the need for participatory versus bureaucratic management.[3]

Shared governance has been defined as a model that allows for decentralized decision-making, increased ownership and accountability in nursing practice, and empowerment within an organization.[5-7] Over the past decade, shared governance has gained popularity because of the rising pressure in nursing and healthcare to become a Magnet-recognized hospital. Ownership and accountability for nursing practice has been elevated as an essential component for nurses and other healthcare providers for improving patient care and is expected in hospitals trying to achieve Magnet recognition.[1,9,10] Becoming a Magnet-recognized hospital has also brought a new set of expectations for leaders and nurses, encouraging them to raise relevant clinical issues and apply systematic approaches to address quality issues such as patient and nursing satisfaction.

Shared governance can be set up in numerous ways within an organization; one size does not fit all. The councilor model typically has various councils, such as practice, education, and quality, and a coordinating council made up of leaders and staff partnering in making decisions.[8,11] The administrative model is similar; however, the organization structures governance to include clinical and administrative focuses. Although the structure is described as being a bit more hierarchal in practice, membership includes both managers and staff in the decision-making process.[8,11] The congressional model provides a venue for staff nurses and leadership to discuss topics and eventually vote on the final decision.[8,11] Some organizations combine aspects of all three models, and others have tried innovative variations. The most important aspect is that there is a structure and process for staff to have input into decisions in order to meet standards of excellence.

For organizations on the Magnet journey, clinical nurse input and shared governance are interwoven throughout the *Magnet Manual*. The manual states, **"Nurses throughout the organization are involved in shared-governance and decision-making structures and processes that establish standards of practice and address opportunities for improvement."**[1] Standard SE1EO* specifically requires organizations to provide two examples of clinical nurses involved in interprofessional decision-making groups at the organizational level and provide outcome data to demonstrate their effectiveness.[1]

Unit-level shared governance works a little differently because units are all different. Some units are small and have few staff members, making it hard to have many unit-level

---

* These standards are based on the 2019 Magnet ® Application Manual. For Magnet Recognition Program® updates and developments, please refer to https://www.nursingworld.org/organizational-programs/magnet/.

councils. Units that are similar, such as labor and delivery, maternity and nursery, and neonatal intensive care units (NICUs), may want to combine efforts into a departmental council structure. Again, the actual structure and processes may differ because there isn't a prescriptive shared governance model that fits every unit, but the end result must provide clinical nurses the ability to have input into management and clinical decisions.

Understanding the differences among authority, accountability, and influence affects the way shared governance is practiced. If these terms aren't clearly defined, staff and leaders can be confused as to who makes what decisions, which eventually leads to discouragement for all participants.

Mercy Medical Center uses the diagram in Exhibit 3.3 to help staff and leaders understand decision-making processes within their hospital. For example, if staff want to begin a performance improvement project affecting only their unit, they may work on the project through their unit-level quality council. However, if staff want to change a policy affecting the entire division, the decision should be made at the division level. If staff want to change a policy affecting the entire organization because it involves multiple disciplines and executive feedback, the policy would most likely be discussed at an interdisciplinary organizational level.

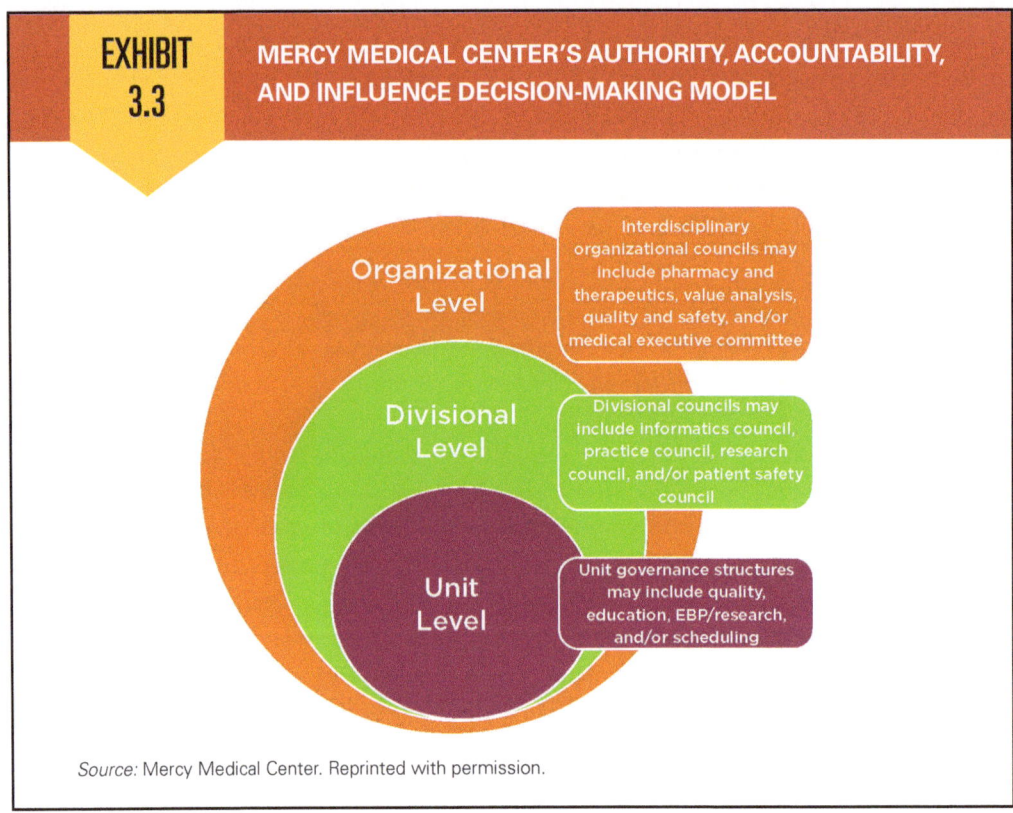

EXHIBIT 3.3

MERCY MEDICAL CENTER'S AUTHORITY, ACCOUNTABILITY, AND INFLUENCE DECISION-MAKING MODEL

Organizational Level

Interdisciplinary organizational councils may include pharmacy and therapeutics, value analysis, quality and safety, and/or medical executive committee

Divisional Level

Divisional councils may include informatics council, practice council, research council, and/or patient safety council

Unit Level

Unit governance structures may include quality, education, EBP/research, and/or scheduling

Source: Mercy Medical Center. Reprinted with permission.

CARE DELIVERY

Organizations need structure and processes by which the responsibility for patient care is assigned and coordinated among members of the nursing staff. The type of care delivery model may differ by unit because of current evidence-based standards, regulatory require- ments, or specific goals. Models used in many organizations include primary nursing, team nursing, and patient- and family-centered nursing. It is important to note that the care delivery model is different from the professional practice model and different from a theory. Table 3.1 describes the difference between a professional practice model, a care delivery model, and the professional practice environment per the *Magnet Manual*.

TABLE 3.1
DIFFERENCES BETWEEN THE PROFESSIONAL PRACTICE MODEL, CARE DELIVERY SYSTEM, AND PROFESSIONAL NURSE PRACTICE ENVIRONMENT

PROFESSIONAL PRACTICE MODEL*	CARE DELIVERY SYSTEM*	NURSING PRACTICE ENVIRONMENT*
A schematic description that describes how nurses practice, collaborate, communicate, and develop professionally.	The structure and processes by which nurses' authority and accountability for patient care are assigned and work is coordi- nated among members of the nursing staff.	Based on theoretical foundations of work, the organizational charac- teristics that facilitate or constrain nursing professional practice.

* The summary descriptions of the terms are based on definitions in the glossary of the *2019 Magnet® Application Manual* (American Nurses Credentialing Center, 2019).

Manthey used five questions to help organizations define their care delivery model[12] (p. 29):

1. Who is responsible for making decisions about patient care?

2. How long do that person's decisions remain in effect?

3. How is the work distributed among staff members: by task or by patient?

4. How is patient care communication handled?

5. How is the whole unit managed?

Organizations on the Magnet journey must define the care delivery system and the impact it has on the delivery of patient care: **"Nurses create patient care delivery systems that delineate the nurses' shared authority and accountability for evidence-based nursing practice, clinical decision-making and outcomes, performance improvement initiatives, and staffing and scheduling processes."**[1] (pg. 40) Organizations are required to describe and demonstrate how they do this through standards EP4EO, EP5, EP6EO, and EP7EO.*

---

* These standards are based on the 2019 Magnet ® Application Manual. For Magnet Recognition Program® updates and developments, please refer to https://www.nursingworld.org/organizational-programs/magnet/.

RECOGNITION, REWARD, AND DEVELOPMENT

For an organization to support high-quality nursing practice, a component of the PPM must include professional growth and development and recognition. Initiatives such as continuing education, career growth, mentoring, and networking, as well as scientific inquiry, are essential in today's environment. The ways in which an organization celebrates and recognizes professional growth and development are equally important.

For those on the Magnet journey, the component of structural empowerment focuses on the need for advancing the profession, valuing the contributions of nurses as well as supporting a culture of lifelong learning.[1] Organizations must show goals in relation to certification achievement and how they met those goals in SE3 and SE4EO. The component of structural empowerment further requires divisions to describe continuing education programs and outcomes, orientation and preceptor programs, and the teaching role of the nurse in SE5, SE6EO, SE7EO, SE8EO, SE9. Standard SE12* asks for organizations to describe and demonstrate how they recognize nursing for meeting strategic goals both individually and as a group.

EXERCISE 3.2	QUICK GAP ANALYSIS ON RECOGNITION, REWARD, AND DEVELOPMENT

1. Does your organization have structures in place to facilitate lifelong learning (e.g., tuition assistance, academic partnerships, continuing education)?

2. Does your organization have a clinical advancement program for nurses?

3. Does your organization have the structures and processes in place to conduct research (e.g., an institutional review board, statistician, library, nurse scientist)?

4. How does your organization recognize nurses both internally and externally?

PROFESSIONAL RELATIONSHIPS

With increasing emphasis on population management and open, transparent communication between disciplines, professional relationships have become paramount for positive patient care outcomes. The Magnet Recognition Program® defines interprofessional team members to include, but not be limited to, social work, psychology, rehabilitation, nutrition, medicine,

---

* These standards are based on the 2019 Magnet ® Application Manual. For Magnet Recognition Program® updates and developments, please refer to https://www.nursingworld.org/organizational-programs/magnet/

and pharmacy.[1] (pg. 40) Therefore, organizations creating a professional practice model need to account for appropriate communication among disciplines and how the communication will be implemented. Mutual respect for achievements of clinical outcomes and strategies to deal with conflict management are also needed within the Professional Relationship domain.

Organizations on the Magnet journey must show a nurse-led (or co-led) collaborative, inter-professional quality improvement activity as well as a patient education activity resulting in positive outcomes in to meet standards EP5, EP6EO,EP7EO and EP8EO.* Embedding profes-sional relationships into the PPM acknowledges the importance of this critical component.

PIECING THE PUZZLE TOGETHER

Bringing your PPM to life in the organization involves three phases (Exhibit 3.4):

1. Development of how you are going to bring the model alive

2. Dissemination of the model, as shown by key responsibilities and accountabilities

3. Enculturation of the model, evidenced by positive outcomes

Within those phases are five steps (illustrated in Exhibit 3.5). The next section will review each of the phases and their respective steps to help bring the PPM to the bedside.

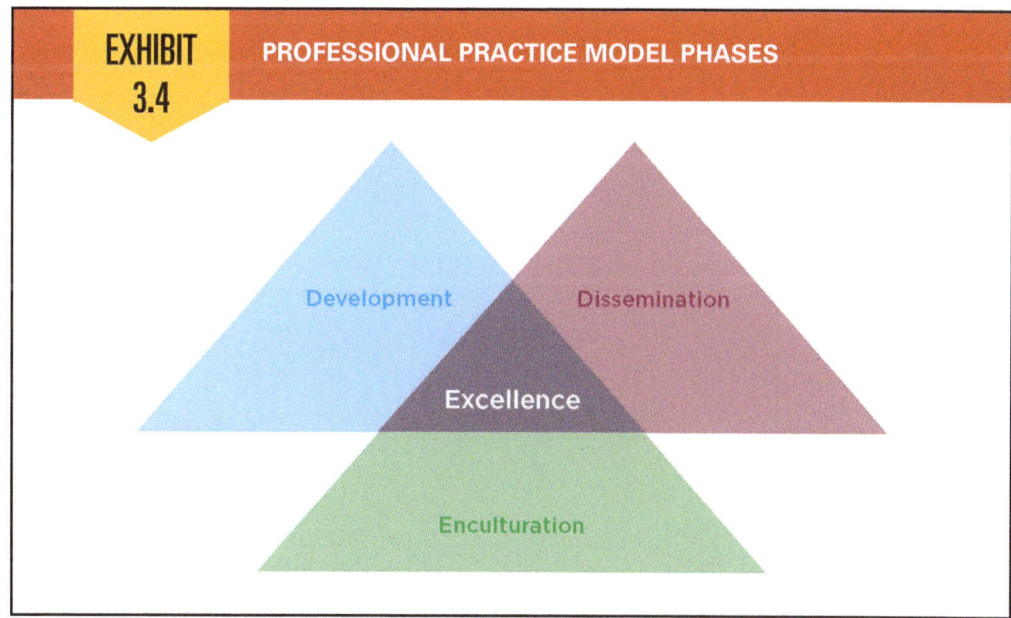

EXHIBIT 3.4 — PROFESSIONAL PRACTICE MODEL PHASES

Development · Dissemination · Excellence · Enculturation

---

*   These standards are based on the 2019 Magnet ® Application Manual. For Magnet Recognition Program® updates and developments, please refer to https://www.nursingworld.org/organizational-programs/magnet/

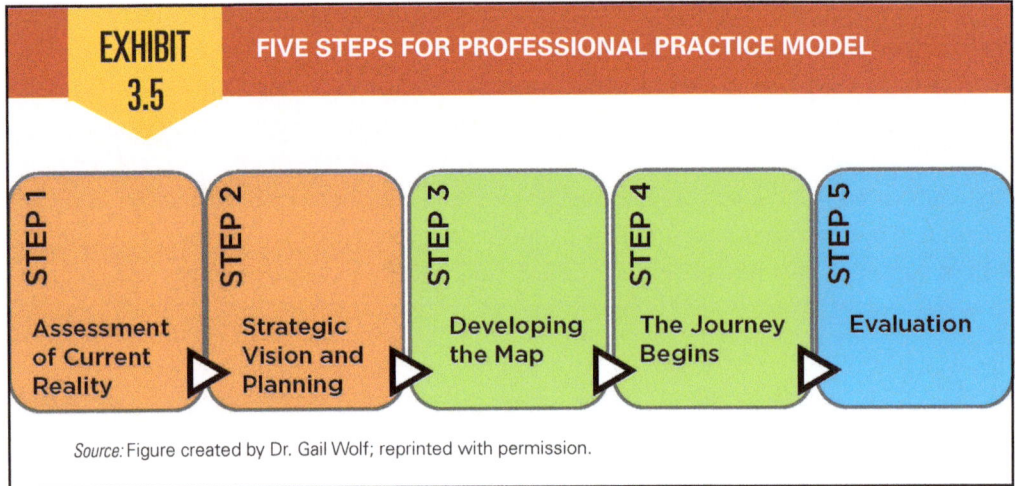

EXHIBIT 3.5

FIVE STEPS FOR PROFESSIONAL PRACTICE MODEL

STEP 1	STEP 2	STEP 3	STEP 4	STEP 5
Assessment of Current Reality	Strategic Vision and Planning	Developing the Map	The Journey Begins	Evaluation

Source: Figure created by Dr. Gail Wolf; reprinted with permission.

Phase 1: Development

Step 1: Assessment of Current Reality

To assess your current reality, it is important to cover specific aspects of internal and external environmental components while still looking into the future. Porter-O'Grady[13] discusses the need to see and incorporate emerging dynamics with the current state so that organizations look further than one or two years ahead.

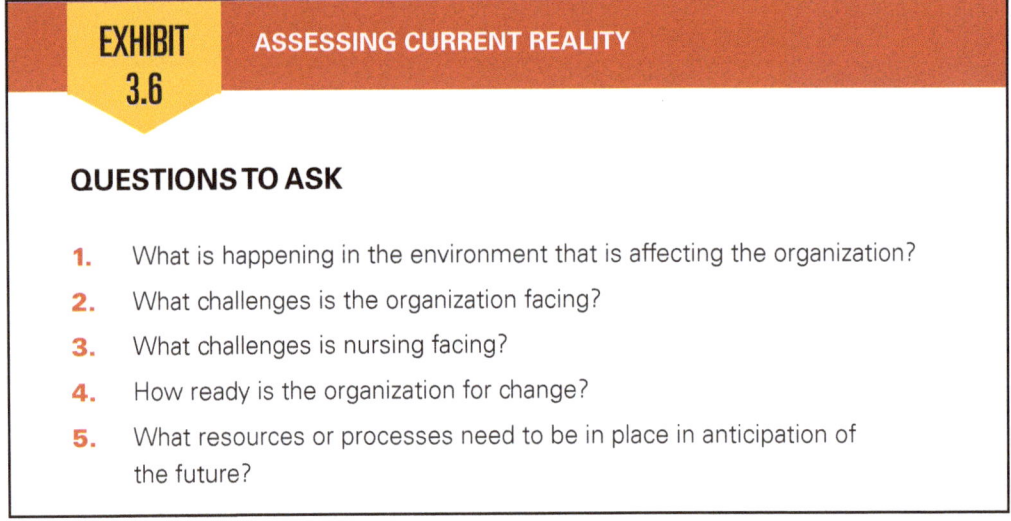

EXHIBIT 3.6

ASSESSING CURRENT REALITY

QUESTIONS TO ASK

1. What is happening in the environment that is affecting the organization?
2. What challenges is the organization facing?
3. What challenges is nursing facing?
4. How ready is the organization for change?
5. What resources or processes need to be in place in anticipation of the future?

External Environments

External components (Table 3.2) include regulatory agencies, benchmarks, new technology, trends, and research as well as the Magnet components. For example, externally the evidence supports improved outcomes with a BSN-prepared workforce. The Institute of Medicine (IOM) report *titled The Future of Nursing: Leading Change, Advancing Health* released in 2010 specifically states as one of its nine recommendations to "increase the proportion of nurses with a baccalaureate degree to 80 percent by 2020"[14] (p. 3). In addition, the Magnet Recognition Program® requires organizations to have not only a completely BSN nursing management team but also a plan on how the organization is going to meet the IOM recommendation of 80% of nurses BSN-prepared by 2020.[1] Knowing this external information, it would be prudent for a nursing team to focus on increasing the number of BSN-prepared nurses in their organization if this recommendation has not already been met.

TABLE 3.2
EXTERNAL ASSESSMENT CATEGORIES

EXTERNAL ASSESSMENT CATEGORIES
Regulatory Agencies
Magnet Program Standards
Trends
New Research Findings
Best Practice Innovations
New Technologies
National Benchmarks
Community Outreach
Healthcare Reform

Another example is the movement towards healthcare reform and improved communication and sharing of information across disciplines as well as healthcare agencies. The *Magnet Manual* states that "Nurses are involved with the design and implementation of technology to enhance the patient experience and nursing practice" (p. 60).[1] Realizing that the norm will be integrated healthcare information systems and a Magnet standard states the need for nurses to be involved in technology, a nursing team should consider putting goals related to information technology and clinical nurse involvement into the strategic plan.

One last example is those items that must be in the strategic plan if applying for Magnet status. Standards EP18EO and EP19EO* specifically emphasize that organizations need to rate above the mean or median the majority of the time for the majority of the units for six nurse-sensitive indicators, including falls with injury, hospital-acquired pressure ulcers stage 2 and above, central line–associated bloodstream infections, catheter-associated urinary tract infections, and two others selected from an approved list in the *Magnet Manual*. When writing a strategic plan, a nursing division could put those outcomes right into the plan to keep the nurses aligned with where the nursing division is headed.

---

* These standards are based on the 2019 Magnet ® Application Manual. For Magnet Recognition Program® updates and developments, please refer to https://www.nursingworld.org/organizational-programs/magnet/

Internal Environment

Another component of assessing current reality is looking at the internal environment (Table 3.3), including the organization's strategic plan, quality data, staff satisfaction, strength of the shared governance model, evidence-based practice, and research, as well as how the organization is perceived internally. It takes both data and qualitative measures to tell the story. Pulling quantitative reports and reviewing areas of opportunity can help focus the team, especially when there are competing priorities.

TABLE 3.3
INTERNAL ASSESSMENT CATEGORIES

INTERNAL ASSESSMENT ITEMS
Quality Data, Nurse-Sensitive Indicators
Dashboards (Certifications, Educational Level, Number of Advancements)
Focus Groups
Patient and Staff Satisfaction Scores
Technology
Financial Reports
Shared Governance Implementation
Human Resources Reports (Turnover and Vacancy)
Evidence-Based Practice and Research
Leadership Development Opportunities
Care Delivery Systems

Step 2: Strategic Vision and Planning

Once the organization completes an external and internal assessment of the environment, realizing the gaps between where the organization could be and where the organization is should be fairly easy. Next, it is time to envision the future (Exhibit 3.7).

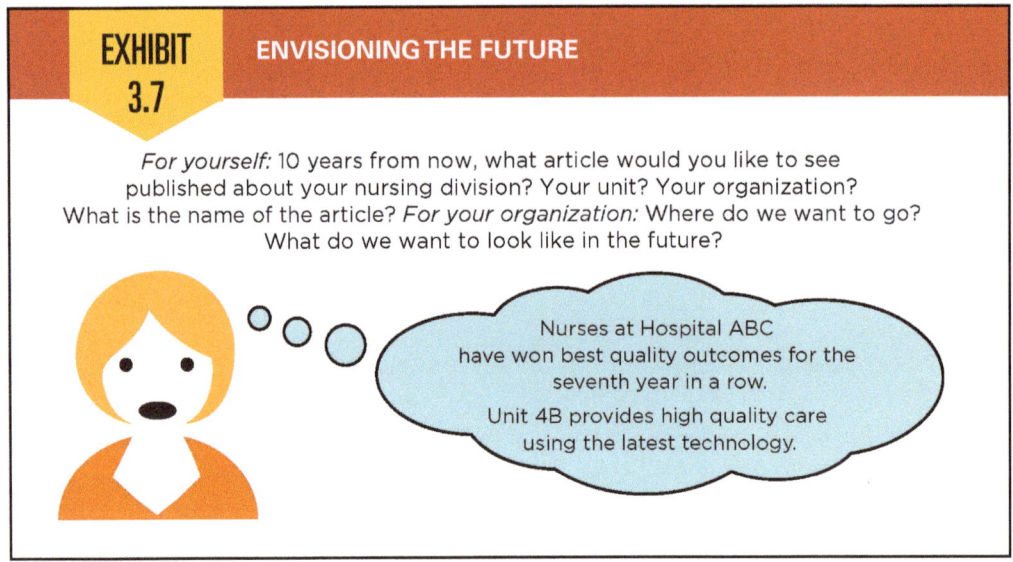

EXHIBIT 3.7 — **ENVISIONING THE FUTURE**

For yourself: 10 years from now, what article would you like to see published about your nursing division? Your unit? Your organization? What is the name of the article? *For your organization:* Where do we want to go? What do we want to look like in the future?

Nurses at Hospital ABC have won best quality outcomes for the seventh year in a row.

Unit 4B provides high quality care using the latest technology.

Envisioning the future provides leaders and staff an opportunity to explore the world of possibilities, which can sometimes showcase more possibilities than resources. Prioritization can help distinguish between what makes it into the strategic plan and what can wait. Remember: success in the past doesn't mean success in the future. Some organizations use focus groups, brainstorming sessions, and workshops to gather ideas from clinical nurses before developing a formal strategic plan. Having clinical nurses involved in the creation of the strategic plan ensures that staff at the point of care have input into the goals and strategies, which could lead to more successful outcomes.

Phase 2: Dissemination

Step 3: Developing the Map

After establishing priorities, it is time to identify goals, time frames, accountabilities, and tactics. Nursing goals should align with the organizational goals, so it is necessary to have the organizational strategic plan when writing the nursing plan.

In the BSN example (Exhibit 3.8), the goal was to achieve 80% BSN staff by increasing the percentage of BSN-prepared nurses every year for the next six years. What would it take for the nurses to meet the goal? How many nurses would need to go back to school

---

EXHIBIT 3.8	STRATEGIC PLAN FRAMEWORK FOR THE BSN EXAMPLE

Professional Practice Model Component: Recognition, Reward, and Development

Goal: Increase percentage of BSN-prepared nurses

Baseline: 48% of nurses currently have a BSN

Measurement: A 5% increase every year for the next six years

Strategies:

- Maintain and support on-site programs for RN to BSN.
- Formalize process to support advanced education.
- Create a formal board with deans and professors from local colleges to meet biannually or annually and discuss changing the environment.
- New hires will be encouraged to enroll in school within two years of hire date to obtain a BSN or higher.
- Provide flexible scheduling for staff wanting to complete BSN.
- Require Clinical IV of the clinical advancement program to have a BSN.

Responsible: Unit shared governance

---

each year? Is the tuition assistance program supportive of staff returning to school? Do you need to change your hiring policy to hire only BSN nurses? How will you communicate any changes that need to happen to meet the goal? Who is accountable for this goal? Nursing management? Human resources?

Standard SE10 a and b * in the *Magnet Manual* describes the need for organizational support in community outreach endeavors.[1] What does this look like in the organization? What kinds of support are in place and what needs to be added? Does the care delivery system encourage community outreach? What types of resources are there for community outreach? Do you need to develop more educational offerings or additional screenings? Are there specific cultural needs in the community that need to be addressed?

Once the goals are established, each goal needs a method of measurement as well as strategies or tactics to meet the goal. When possible, it is good to include baseline data as well as who is accountable for the outcomes. Exhibit 3.8 describes the key aspects needed to build the strategic plan framework.

Step 4: The Journey Begins

It is now time to operationalize all components into practice. This step takes a lot of energy, communication, and reinforcement. There are many ways to bring your PPM and your strategic plan to life within the organization. Strategies can include incorporating the items in newsletters, agendas, job descriptions, peer review, workshops, and inservices. Communication methods such as email, posters, bulletin boards, flyers, screen savers, and badge-holder cards can keep the strategies visually in front of the staff. The Chief Nursing Officer could reinforce strategies through presentations at the board or executive level. Last, both the PPM and the strategic plan documents are needed for Magnet recognition, so it is important for staff to know and understand both concepts.[1]

One tool used at Mercy Medical Center was the one-page dashboard. The dashboard helped councils, staff, leaders, and ancillary departments know where the nursing division was focused. Exhibit 3.9 is their example of a dashboard.

Another way the organization disseminated the information was by aligning meeting agendas to the PPM and strategic plan categories. Having the components of the PPM right on the agenda can help the nurses focus on key strategic initiatives. Redesigning job descriptions to match your PPM is another way to bring it alive in the organization. When writing your newsletters or annual report, your organization could link the articles back to the strategic plan, the PPM, or both. Describing the PPM and strategic plan during orientation

---

* These standards are based on the 2019 Magnet ® Application Manual. For Magnet Recognition Program® updates and developments, please refer to https://www.nursingworld.org/organizational-programs/magnet/

EXHIBIT 3.9	MERCY MEDICAL CENTER DASHBOARD

Nursing Strategic Plan Abbreviated Version
FY12–FY16

COLLABORATIVE CARE PRACTICE	TRANSFORMATIONAL LEADERSHIP	CULTURE	EVIDENCE, RESEARCH, AND INNOVATION	PROFESSIONAL GROWTH AND DEVELOPMENT
Patient- and Family-Centered Care	Business of Healthcare	Community Outreach	Evidence-Based Practice	Clinical Ladder
Collaboration/Teamwork Multiple Disciplines	Leadership Development	Magnet Status	Research	Charge Nurse and Preceptor Workshop
Quality Measures	Shared Governance	Peer Review	Innovation in Practice	National Certifications and Advanced Degrees
Electronic Health Record and Meaningful Use		Work/Life Balance	Presentations and Publications	NST Development
Bunting Move				

Source: Stacey Brull; Mercy Medical Center, reprinted with permission.

is another way to show new employees the direction of the nursing division. The point is to make sure the PPM and strategic plan are fully integrated into daily operations.

CASE STUDY: INTEGRATING THE PPM INTO PRACTICE

In 2014, the Mercy Medical Center nursing leadership team and 60 nurses met for a strategic planning workshop to review and revise the then-current PPM. At that workshop, participants identified the need to consolidate their model and remove parts that they didn't see in the future. For example, they felt they did not need to have a separate section focused on recruitment and retention because all of their vacancies had been filled with a waiting list. Instead, they wanted to focus more time on professional growth and development because they felt that would keep nurses at Mercy and at the bedside. Another area the team felt was important was combining care delivery with interprofessional relationships because interdisciplinary collaboration is so critical in the new healthcare reform and pay-for-performance models.

Once the PPM was finalized (see Exhibit 3.10), the same group of nurses and nurse leaders discussed specific goals to fit each of the PPM components. For example, one goal under Mercy's PPM component of Transformational Leadership is having leaders recognized and known as transformational.

EXHIBIT
3.10

MERCY MEDICAL CENTER'S 2014 PPM REVISED WITH
STAFF INPUT

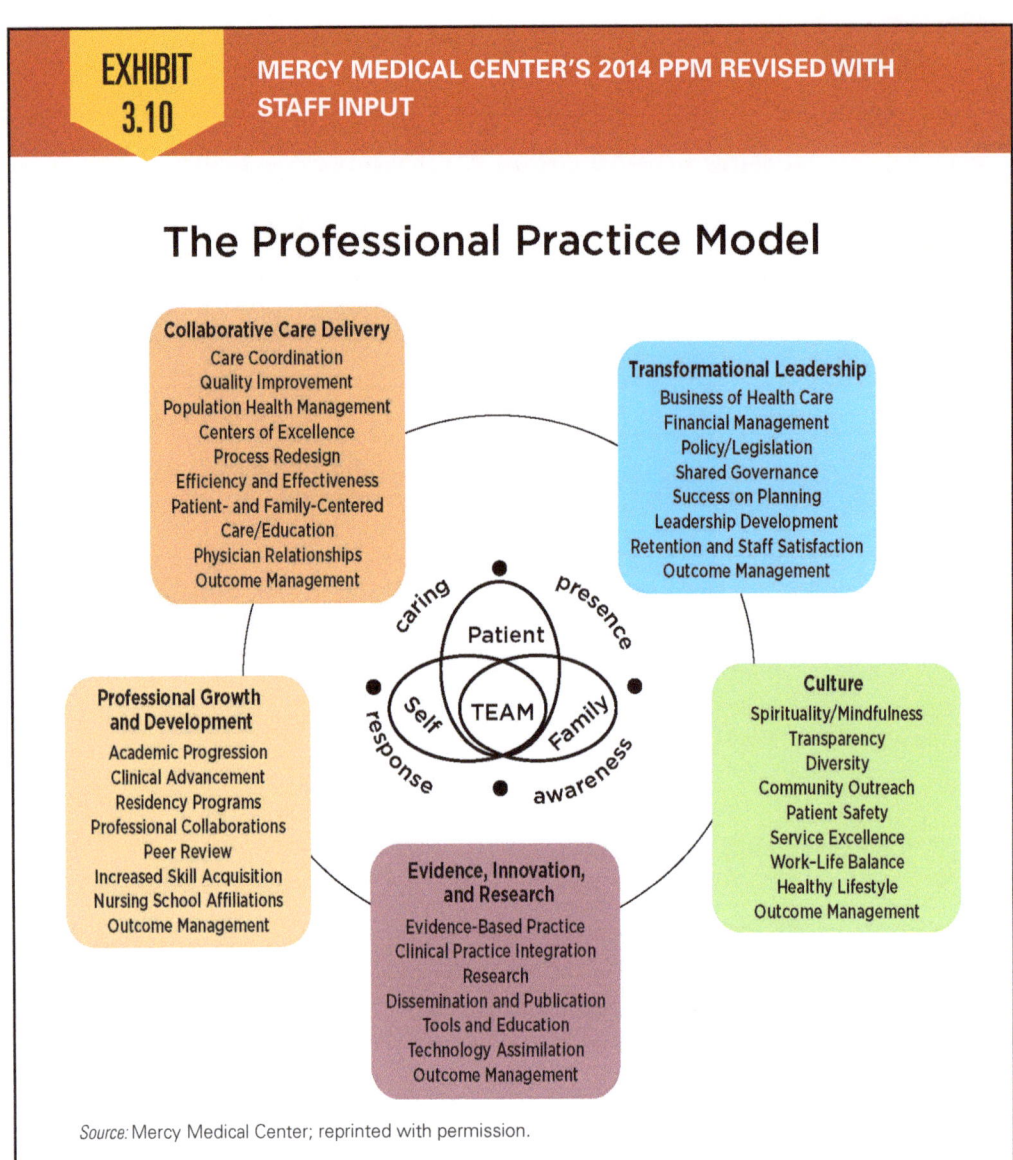

The Professional Practice Model

Collaborative Care Delivery
Care Coordination
Quality Improvement
Population Health Management
Centers of Excellence
Process Redesign
Efficiency and Effectiveness
Patient- and Family-Centered
Care/Education
Physician Relationships
Outcome Management

Transformational Leadership
Business of Health Care
Financial Management
Policy/Legislation
Shared Governance
Success on Planning
Leadership Development
Retention and Staff Satisfaction
Outcome Management

**Professional Growth
and Development**
Academic Progression
Clinical Advancement
Residency Programs
Professional Collaborations
Peer Review
Increased Skill Acquisition
Nursing School Affiliations
Outcome Management

Culture
Spirituality/Mindfulness
Transparency
Diversity
Community Outreach
Patient Safety
Service Excellence
Work-Life Balance
Healthy Lifestyle
Outcome Management

**Evidence, Innovation,
and Research**
Evidence-Based Practice
Clinical Practice Integration
Research
Dissemination and Publication
Tools and Education
Technology Assimilation
Outcome Management

caring · presence · Patient · Self · TEAM · Family · response · awareness

Source: Mercy Medical Center; reprinted with permission.

Goal 2: Leaders are recognized and known as transformational.

One of the strategies to meet this goal was to increase leadership and staff participation in professional organizations. Each strategy must have measurable outcomes and specific tactics to meet those outcomes. Tactics can change throughout the year(s) as needed; however, the ultimate goal is to meet the measurable outcome defined. A second example shows a goal to have nurses dedicated to professional development and lifelong learning. One of the strategies for this goal is to strengthen teaching methods to be learner-centered. Again, the example shows tactics, outcomes, and accountability (Exhibit 3.11).

GOAL 1: Nurses are dedicated to professional development and lifelong learning.

Strategy	Measurable Outcome	Tactics	Coordinator	Accountable
Strengthening our teaching strategies to be learner centered	5 new innovative teaching strategies	• Utilize online learning capabilities, social media and other instructional design methodologies. • Increase use of multimodal strategies such as simulation, gamification. • Encourage formal classes on teaching methods for staff and leaders. • Mentor staff nurses in the art of presenting. • Increase the amount of just-in-time training at the unit level. • Look for opportunities to decrease costs due to education. • Continue using nursing spectrum online continuing education module. • Develop a database that tracks all nursing continuing education programs with a focus on outcomes. • Develop outcome measures and a formal education plan prior to teaching • Utilize the nursing needs assessment tool to develop educational opportunities that are meaningful to the staff.	Sr. Director For Education	Education Council Center for Clinical Excellence

GOAL 2: Leaders are recognized and known as transformational.

Strategy	Measurable Outcomes	Tactics	Coordinator	Accountable
Increase leadership and staff participation in professional and/or political organizations at the local, state, or national level	15 leadership officers and taskforce members 35% of clinical nurses as members 7 leaders participate on a board by 2016	• Recognize and reward nursing leaders who actively participate in professional/political organizations. • Attend nursing advocacy events locally and/or nationally. • Send staff and leaders to health policy workshops and/or classes. • Add an "In the News" section as a standing agenda item on all meeting agendas. (ATONE, WIFE, I OM, AACHEN, HI, CMS, HRSA, CAHRA, etc.). Incorporate professional/political organization involvement into Moments of Excellence and MercyCares Newsletter. • Provide opportunities for leaders and clinical nurses to be engaged through shadowing opportunities, networking or attending a meeting.	Chief Nursing Officer	Professional Practice Council Nursing Leadership

Source: Mercy Medical Center; reprinted with permission.

TABLE 3.4
EVIDENCE, RESEARCH, AND INNOVATION

STRATEGY	OUTCOME	JAN	FEB	MAR	APR	MAY	JUN	JULY	AUG	SEP	OCT	NOV	DEC
Disseminate results of research internally and externally	10 peer-reviewed abstract presentations; 4 publications submitted and 2 accepted per year												

Step 5: Evaluation

Organizations often ask, "How do we know our PPM and strategic plan are working?" Using a dashboard helps; ensuring that the entire division visits the strategic plan dashboard on a quarterly basis is essential. Having the responsible parties bring their updated reports and statistics to a divisional meeting helps keep the focus alive and in front of key stakeholders.

Another way to evaluate the effectiveness of your strategic plan is to use it to write your Magnet stories. Did you write the correct measurements and goals to have empirical outcome stories? Using Mercy Medical Center again, we can look at their Magnet example for national certifications and see that they met the goal (Exhibit 3.12).

CONCLUSION

The PPM and the strategic plan play a vital role in moving a nursing division along the path toward excellence. Bringing clinical nurses into the design, development, implementation, and evaluation of the PPM and the nursing strategic plan is essential to not only meet Magnet Recognition Program® standards but also ensure accountability and successful outcomes. Although developing the PPM and strategic plan takes time and resources, if both are built correctly, they will define the direction the division is headed and provide a much-needed roadmap for everyone involved in the journey.

The authors would like to gratefully acknowledge the contributions of Dr. Stacy Brull and Dr. Gail Wolf to this section.

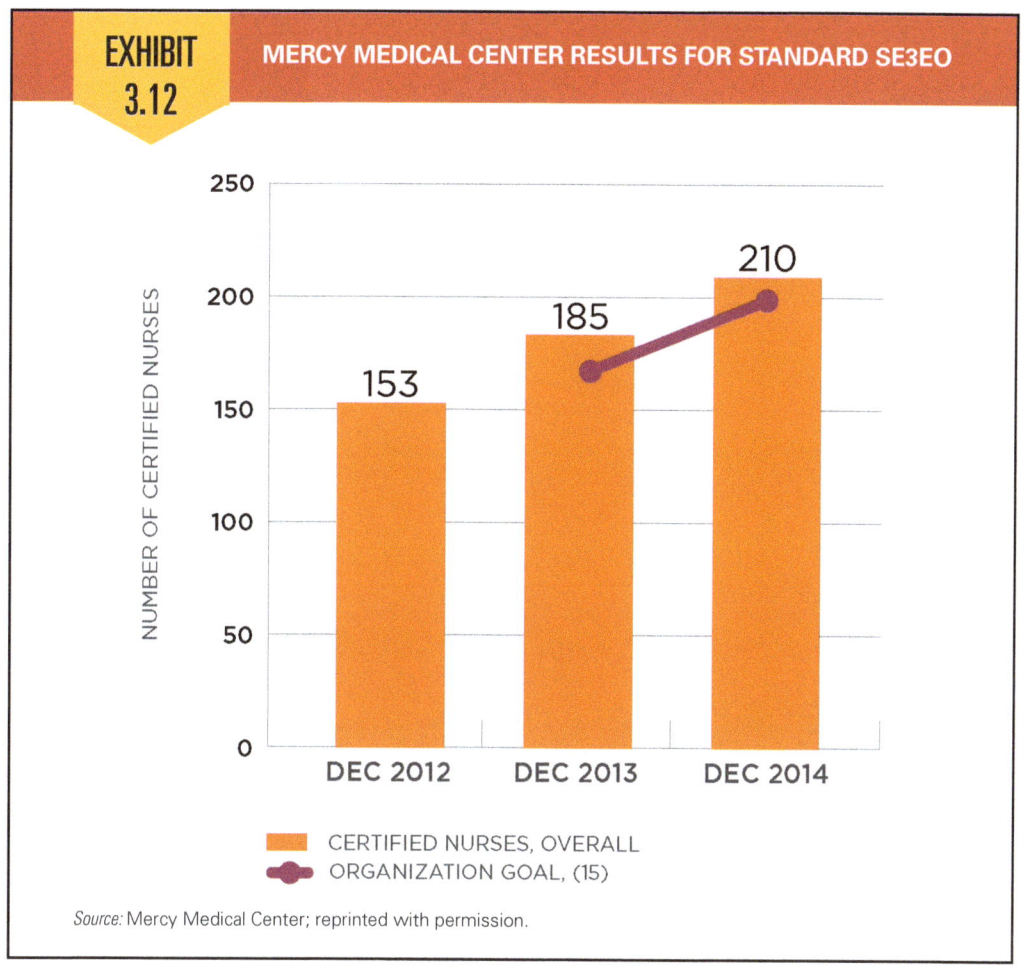

EXHIBIT 3.12

NUMBER OF CERTIFIED NURSES

210
185
153

DEC 2012   DEC 2013   DEC 2014

CERTIFIED NURSES, OVERALL
ORGANIZATION GOAL, (15)

Source: Mercy Medical Center; reprinted with permission.

REFERENCES

1. American Nurses Credentialing Center. (2019). 2019 Magnet application manual. Silver Spring, MD.: Author.

2. Mensik, J. S. (2013). The importance of professional practice models in nurse staffing. *Nurse Leader, 11*(4), 65–68.

3. Hoffart, N., & Woods, C. Q. (1996). Elements of a nursing professional practice model. *Journal of Professional Nursing, 12*(6), 354–364.

4. Wolf, G., Aukerman, M., & Boland, S. (1999). *The transformational model for professional practice in health care organizations.* Pittsburg: The Beckwith Institute for Innovation in Nursing: UMPC Health System.

5. Porter-O'Grady, T. (2001). Is shared governance still relevant? *Journal of Nursing Administration, 31*(10), 468–473.

6. Williamson, T. (2005). Work-based learning: A leadership development example from an action research study of shared governance implementation. *Journal of Nursing Management, 13*(6), 490–499.

7. Waddell, A. W. (2009). Cultivating quality: Shared governance supports evidence-based practice. *AJN The American Journal of Nursing, 109*(11), 53–57

8. Hess, R. G., Jr. (2011). Slicing and dicing shared governance: In and around the numbers. *Nursing Administration Quarterly, 35*(3), 235–241.

9. American Nurses Credentialing Center. (2008). *Magnet Recognition Program® Manual.* Silver Spring, MD: Author.

10. Institute of Medicine. (2006*). The future of nursing: Leading change, advancing health.* Institute of Medicine and Robert Wood Johnson Foundation.

11. Porter-O'Grady, T. (1992). *Implementing shared governance: Creating a professional organization.* St. Louis, MO: Mosby Year Book.

12. Manthey, M. (1991). Delivery systems and practice models: A dynamic balance. *Nursing Management, 22*(1), 28–30.

13. Porter-O'Grady, T. (2010). A new age for practice: Creating the framework for evidence. In K. Malloch & T. Porter-O'Grady (Eds.), *Introduction to evidence-based practice in nursing and health care* (pp. 1–29). Sudbury, MA: Jones and Bartlett.

14. Institute of Medicine. (2010). *The future of nursing: Leading change, advancing health.* (p 3). Institute of Medicine and Robert Wood Johnson Foundation.

RECOGNIZING DEVELOPMENTAL LEVELS

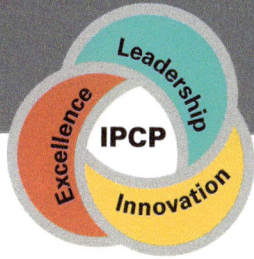

RECOGNIZING DEVELOPMENTAL LEVELS

Trying to change before you're ready isn't likely to be productive. For example, most New Year's resolutions don't last because people spring into action without being prepared for the work it's going to take. Forcing change based on the calendar, rather than a true readiness to transform, can be a setup for failure.

—Amy Morin

The need for high-performing teams isn't a new concept in organizational development. Nelson and Burns[1] discuss the need for specific conditions within a workplace that lead to high-performing units, teams, and individuals. Their model consists of four developmental stages, starting with the reactive stage and moving toward high performance.

The four developmental levels are (1) reactive, (2) responsive, (3) proactive, and (4) high performing. These four levels can be used to evaluate units, teams, organizations, or individuals. Depending on what is being measured, one may find different developmental levels within the same unit, as well as different developmental levels between employees. For example, a unit may be proactive in community service but responsive in evidence-based practice; likewise, a unit may include some personnel functioning at a reactive level while others demonstrate proactive behaviors. Wolf and colleagues[2] wrote an article describing each of the levels based on the Magnet® standards to help nurses evaluate their unit, organization, or team. This step will describe each level. Following each description, a case study will demonstrate that particular level as well as questions to think about in connection to the Magnet standards.

RECOMMENDED READING

Vuurberg, G., Vos, J. A. M., Christoph, L. H., & de Vos, R. (2019). The effectiveness of interprofessional classroom-based education in medical curricula: A systematic review. *Journal of Interprofessional Education & Practice*, 15, 157–167. DOI: 10.1016/j.xjep.2019.01.007

Wolf, G., Finlayson, S., Hayden, M., Hoolahan, S., & Mazzoccoli, A. (2014). The developmental levels in achieving Magnet designation, part 1. *Journal of Nursing Administration*, *44*(3): 136–141.

Wolf, G., Finlayson, S., Hayden, M., Hoolahan, S., & Mazzoccoli, A. (2014). The developmental levels in achieving Magnet designation, part 2. *Journal of Nursing Administration*, *44*(4): 196–200.

EXHIBIT 4.1

DEVELOPMENTAL STAGES LEADING TOWARD HIGH PERFORMANCE

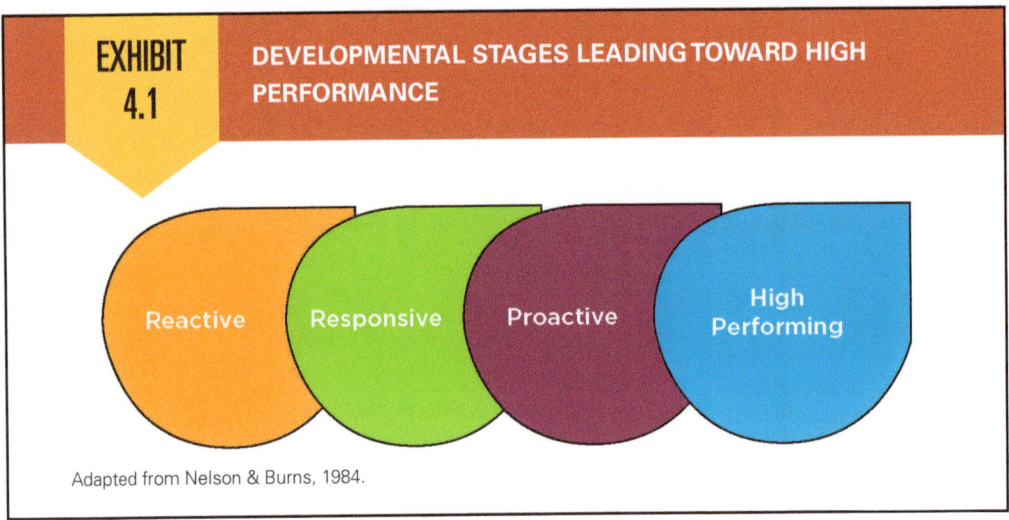

Reactive   Responsive   Proactive   High Performing

Adapted from Nelson & Burns, 1984.

OVERVIEW OF THE FOUR DEVELOPMENTAL LEVELS

1. **Reactive**: A unit or organization does not begin at a reactive level. This developmental level occurs because there is a mismatch between the employees and the leader's style, which is typically either too punitive or too passive. Units, organizations, and people in a reactive phase tend to focus on the past, often with a victim mentality of "us" versus "them." Nelson and Burns describe reactive areas as having fragmented

structures, punitive changes, and force-fed communication.[1] Management tends to be top-down (or passive) and often strongly negative toward informal leaders, which undermine progress and intimidates coworkers. Cliques are common in this environment. There is little interest in taking risks for fear of punishment, leading to a blaming culture.[2]

2. **Responsive**: Units, organizations, and people in a responsive framework are fairly stable. Everyone works together relatively well and is focused on the present. Leadership has moved from punitive or passive to motivating, typically through rewarding and recognizing high performance.[1] A hierarchal structure is still in place, though with increased coordination and cohesiveness. Overall, the environment feels healthy. Everyone follows the rules and works to improve performance and outcomes.

3. **Proactive**: Units, organizations, and people in a proactive framework are looking toward the future. Nelson and Burns state that in a proactive framework the future is something that can be changed versus a place where you remain stable.[1] There is trust between staff and leadership, and the focus is on the greater good for the division, the organization, or both.[2] Leaders are more strategic and act systematically. Results are aligned with strategic goals, and employees are motivated by what they contribute. Magnet organizations should be at minimum in a proactive framework with some at the high-performing stage.

4. **High Performing**: Units, organizations, and people functioning at a high-performing stage see endless possibilities within the nursing division and the organization as well as the larger community, profession, or environment. High-performing areas make contributions both internally and externally. They see their role as change agents for the greater good of society.[1] Employees are empowered to transform their environment. The focus is on excellence and working through networks and relationships.

TABLE 4.1
DIMENSIONS OF THE FOUR STAGES

FRAMEWORK	REACTIVE	RESPONSIVE	PROACTIVE	HIGH-PERFORMING
Time Frame	Past	Present	Future	Endless
Perspective	Self	Team	Organization	Culture
Development	Survival	Cohesion	Accommodating	Transformational
Leadership	Enforcing	Coaching	Purposing	Empowering

Partially adapted from Nelson & Burns, 1984.

OPERATIONALIZING THE THEORY

The underlying theory of this four-stage model of organizational development can be better understood in terms of its application in practice settings. The rest of Step 4 offers a case study of each developmental level:

- Case Study 1: Moving from reactive to responsive

- Case Study 2: Moving from responsive to proactive

- Case Study 3: Moving from proactive to higher performing

- Case Study 4: Arriving as high-performing organization

EXHIBIT 4.2   **CASE STUDY 1: CASE STUDY OF A REACTIVE UNIT**

Angela Montgomery was hired as a clinical nurse on C4. From past hospital experience, she understood the importance of shared governance on patient outcomes. She was eager to learn how C4 incorporated shared governance into unit operations.

It became clear there was an absence of shared governance on C4 as evidenced by decision-making being done primarily at the top. The unit's patient satisfaction scores were in the low percentiles, and the unit had five falls, including two with an injury, in the past week. Angela believed she could promote the positive behaviors and practices needed to improve these scores through a shared governance model. She asked her manager if she could try to start shared governance, and her manager wished her good luck.

Angela asked for volunteers from C4 to help bring shared governance to the unit. Denise Bolinski and Trent Dooble, C4 registered nurses, told Angela they would help her get the process started. Angela was thrilled by their interest and enthusiasm. The three set up a meeting time, agenda, and sign-up sheet.

On the meeting day, Angela looked at the sign-in sheet posted in the staff break room. No RNs had signed up to participate in the meeting. Angela expressed her concern to Denise and Trent. She asked why no RNs had signed up to attend the meeting. Angela explained that C4 staff had a history of rejecting change. Trent went on to say that a few of the nurses did not really promote a lot of progress on the unit because they liked it the way it had always been, and some are were afraid of the manager, who "called the shots." The manager didn't attend the meeting. Angela wasn't sure what she needed to do to improve the situation other than look for another job at another hospital.

Reviewing the Case Study of a Reactive Unit

Accurately identifying a developmental level can be tricky. The example above demonstrates a lot of reactive elements. For example, decision-making was done primarily at the top. Quality indicators and patient satisfaction scores were substandard. The nurses showed little enthusiasm to engage in shared governance. The two nurses who did volunteer said that staff were afraid of the manager. All of these statements appear to indicate a reactive unit. Ask yourself, what could be done to turn the unit around? More importantly, what aspects of Magnet are missing?

The *2019 Magnet Application Manual* (hereafter *Magnet Manual*) states the following:[3]

- "Nurses throughout the organization are involved in shared governance, decision-making structures and processes that establish standards of practice and address opportunities for improvement." (p. 25)

- "Magnet organizations demonstrate outcome measures that generally outperform the benchmark statistic of the national database used in patient- and nurse-sensitive indicators." (p. 41)

- "The CNO should be visible and accessible and should communicate effectively in an environment of mutual respect. As a result, nurses throughout the organization should perceive that their voices are heard, their input is valued, and their practice is supported." (p. 20)

Therefore, according to the developmental level tool, this unit would not meet Magnet standards in relation to transformational leadership, structural empowerment, or exemplary professional practice.

Moving from Reactive to Responsive

The unit in the case study needs to begin using principles of change management to move from reactive to responsive. These principles include the need to establish a sense of urgency, create and communicate a vision, empower others to act on the vision, and create short-term wins.[4] The manager begins the process by clarifying goals and developing trust with the staff. Involving staff in solving problems before they occur and planning specific actions with accountability are two additional steps to successful change. Situational-leadership principles are very helpful in a reactive phase. Situational leadership provides the leader flexibility to adapt his or her style based on the knowledge and experience of the individual or the situation.[5] Hershey and Blanchard[5] describe the leadership behaviors as telling, selling, participating, and delegating.

Sometimes, even when a manager has all the right intentions, he or she may still have trouble developing a unit. In this scenario, the Chief Nursing Officer may need to get involved. The Chief Nursing Officer (CNO) has ultimate accountability and responsibility for ensuring the organization and all units within the organization are performing at proactive or high-performing levels in order to be recognized as a Magnet organization. Therefore, the CNO must help the staff and the leadership team develop strategies to achieve further development. This intervention may be in the form of a workshop or a series of workshops, or it may involve using a facilitator to engage the staff in developing a plan based on unit-level data and metrics. If a unit is in a reactive state, it is unlikely that critical data points such as patient satisfaction, staff satisfaction, and quality indicators outperform the organizational mean the majority of the time. Data are a powerful illustration for staff to see the quality of care they provide.

Managing "Royalty"

A common challenge in moving from reactive to responsive and sometimes from responsive to proactive is managing "royalty" or bullies. Classically these are strong, clinically competent nurses who use their expert power to achieve personal gain rather than to improve the unit or organization. They typically have a following and often intimidate less experienced colleagues to retain power. It is critical for the leader to manage these individuals by not tolerating their negative behavior and by not enabling them. If these nurses are in key informal or formal leadership positions, rethinking the structure and leadership roles on the unit is critical. Breaking up cliques by changing committee structures or rotating new staff into important positions will start to shift the power. The leader will also need to have crucial conversations with these nurses specifically discussing the expected changes in their behavior.

EXHIBIT 4.3   **CLUES TO ENABLING "ROYALTY"**

Are you wondering if you enable your royalty? Ask yourself the following questions:

1. Are they in charge of the schedule?
2. Are they the "go-to" people or in charge often?
3. Do they chair a council or run key meetings?
4. Do you give them excellent or high-performing performance evaluations?
5. Have they been promoted on a clinical advancement program?

If you answered yes to any of these questions, you may be creating a sense of power for your kings and queens.

Evaluation of Case Study 1

It is important to continually evaluate whether the unit, the organization, or an individual is continuing to develop. Wolf and colleagues describe various situations on the reactive to high-performing continuum to help leaders and staff understand where they may be in terms of Magnet Recognition Program® standards. Using the gap analysis tool provided by Wolf and colleagues[2] (p. 101) can illustrate how the unit is progressing.

In the case study of the reactive unit, shared governance and professional engagement appear to be reactive. As staff become more involved in decisions on their unit and as quality indicators improve, the unit will slowly begin to feel more healthy, which will begin the transition from reactive to responsive.

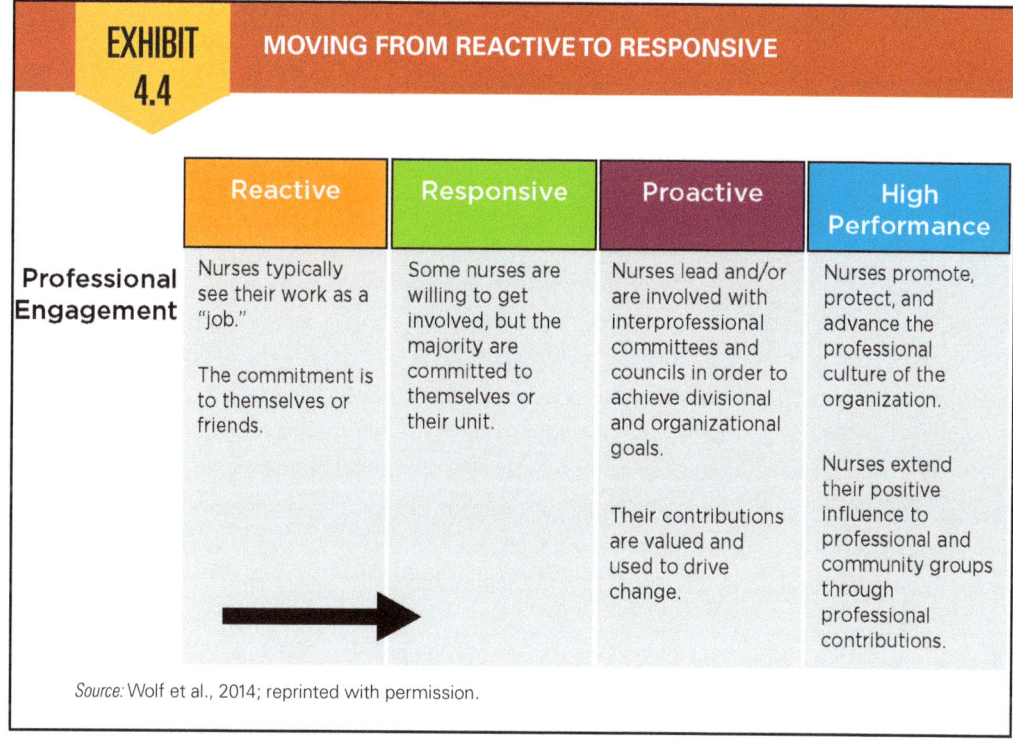

EXHIBIT 4.4 — MOVING FROM REACTIVE TO RESPONSIVE

	Reactive	Responsive	Proactive	High Performance
Professional Engagement	Nurses typically see their work as a "job." The commitment is to themselves or friends.	Some nurses are willing to get involved, but the majority are committed to themselves or their unit.	Nurses lead and/or are involved with interprofessional committees and councils in order to achieve divisional and organizational goals. Their contributions are valued and used to drive change.	Nurses promote, protect, and advance the professional culture of the organization. Nurses extend their positive influence to professional and community groups through professional contributions.

Source: Wolf et al., 2014; reprinted with permission.

Reviewing the Case Study of a Responsive Unit

Tower 4 (Exhibit 4.5) exemplifies a responsive unit as evidenced by their acceptance of being stable. The nurses did not show any interest in going above and beyond what was expected of them. Realizing there was a reward if they improved their scores provided them with the motivation to work on the issue. The nurses appear to work well together and are known for their teamwork and shared governance system. They also set goals and achieve them. Their lack of enthusiasm or self-drive to conduct research or take their idea hospital-wide also highlights a responsive unit.

Using the developmental level tool created by Wolf and colleagues,[2] you can see that this unit would not meet Magnet standards in relation to exemplary professional practice or new knowledge and innovations.

The *Magnet Manual* states the following:[3]

- "Magnet nurses partner with patients, families, support systems, and interprofessional teams to positively impact patient care and outcomes." (p. 40)

- "Magnet-recognized organizations conscientiously integrate evidence-based practice and research into clinical and operational processes." (p. 59)

- "Innovations in patient care, nursing, and the practice environment are the hallmark of organizations receiving Magnet recognition." (p. 60)

Moving From Responsive to Proactive

One of the ways to move from responsive to proactive is to incorporate both individual and unit short- and long-range goals and tie them back to the organizational and nursing strategic plan. Moving from unit-specific initiatives to divisional initiatives starts the evolution toward a more proactive unit.

In a responsive setting, the leader still works under a controlled framework. Using transformational leadership components will begin to move a unit toward proactive. Dr. Bruce Avolio and colleagues[6] describe the components of a transformational leader to be (1) idealized influence, (2) intellectual stimulation, (3) individualized consideration, and (4) inspirational motivation. A quick definition of each component will help clarify why this specific switch in leadership style is so critical to unit development.

A leader using idealized influence leads by example, is visionary, has charisma, and is a role model for what can be versus what is. Using intellectual stimulation, the leader encourages creativity, problem-solving, and innovation. As a coach and mentor to staff, the leader exhibits individualized consideration, and by promoting excitement, enthusiasm, and positive energy, the leader inspires motivation to continuously improve and excel.

Evaluation of Case Study 2

It is important to continually evaluate whether the unit, the organization, or the individual is moving in the right direction. Using the tool provided by Wolf and colleagues,[2] one can easily see how the unit in the case study is in a responsive state in terms of exemplary professional

The fourth-floor Med/Surg unit (Tower 4) of Healthy Hospital is known for shared governance. Staff is involved in many of the decisions on the unit. Recently, the quality council on the unit received patient satisfaction scores and saw their scores had declined regarding explanation of new medicines.

A group of staff nurses went to the literature to see if there were any articles describing best practices to improve their scores. Naomi Butler, RN, found a few articles showcasing the teach-back method to improve patient satisfaction scores. Naomi brought this information back to the unit, which began implementing the new practice. The following quarter, the unit saw their percentile rankings go from 56% to 75%. The unit knew that because their scores improved so much, they were surely going to win the free lunch contest.

After the lunch, the CNO asked if the staff would be interested in leading a hospital-wide research study on patient satisfaction. A few people acted interested, but no one volunteered to lead the potential study; therefore, it never happened. At the next shared governance meeting, Naomi stated that their scores had remained stable and there were not any new quality issues on the unit.

	Reactive	Responsive	Proactive	High Performance
Research	Research is not strongly valued.	Nurses may participate in research projects, but they rarely initiate research.	Nurses generate research and apply research to their practice.	Nurses are actively involved in generating and disseminating research on a national or international level.

Source: Wolf et al., 2014; reprinted with permission.

practice and new knowledge and innovation. As the leadership pushes the staff to focus on larger, more divisional goals, more emphasis will be on interprofessional collaboration as well as how staff contribute to the organization and the profession of nursing as a whole.

Reviewing the Case Study of a Proactive Unit

The ability of the nurses on this unit to engage in a research study shows how much the unit and the Division of Nursing support empowerment and autonomy. The collaboration between the physicians and the nurses demonstrates an environment supportive of nurses leading interdisciplinary teams to improve the quality of care. The study also demonstrates nurses engaged in their professional organizations and understanding the need to incorporate national standards and guidelines into practice. One can easily ascertain that this unit is performing at a proactive level. When reading the case study, one can feel the high energy of the nurses, the excitement, and the healthy collaboration between disciplines. This unit would meet the Magnet standards of excellence.

The *Magnet Manual* states the following:[3]

- "The autonomous nurse provides care based on the unique needs and attributes of the patient and their family, support system, or both." (p. 50)

- "Nurses create patient care delivery systems that delineate the nurses' shared authority and accountability for evidence-based nursing practice, clinical decision-making and outcomes, performance improvement initiative, and staff and scheduling processes." (p. 50)

- "Nurses collaborate with other disciplines to ensure that care is comprehensive, coordinated, and monitored for effectiveness through the quality improvement model."(p. 51).

Moving From Proactive to High Performing

Being a proactive nurse, unit, or organization does meet Magnet standards. Therefore, the difference between proactive and high-performing levels revolves more around who is involved and how they are involved. Proactive performance focuses on the contributions to the nursing division as a whole, whereas the focus for high performance shifts to the overall organization and nursing community at large. Proactive-level units or nurses tend to identify and implement innovative solutions, whereas high-performing units or nurses tend to identify, develop, implement, and disseminate innovative solutions though publications and presentations.[2]

EXHIBIT
4.7

CASE STUDY 3: A PROACTIVE UNIT

Unit 6 South has staff attending all of the Divisional Council meetings regularly, including the Quality, Education, and Practice Councils. In the past year, the 6 South staff have increased their patient satisfaction scores from the 80th percentile to the 95th percentile, conducted an evidence-based-practice project resulting in a decreased length of stay for patients undergoing orthopedic surgery, and promoted eight staff on the clinical advancement program.

More recently, a group of staff discussed starting a research study involving the use of alternative postoperative antinausea products for patients. The staff completed a literature review on the topic. Knowing this would be a multidisciplinary project, Susie, the Chair of the Research Council for the Division and a Clinical Nurse IV on the orthopedic unit, met with her manager and the Chair of Orthopedics. Dr. Hinter, Chair of Orthopedic Surgery, thought the study would need to include anesthesiology as well as the post-anesthesia unit. A second meeting was called two weeks later with all the suggested stakeholders as well as the Director of Nursing Perioperative Services and the Director of Medical Surgical Nursing. Susie asked Dr. Hinter if he would like to be a principal investigator on the study, and Dr. Hinter agreed to support the study in any way he could. The study was approved by the institutional review board and the team began the work.

The research study took six months to complete, and the results showed that using alternative methods to decrease nausea and vomiting in postoperative orthopedic patients worked and patients preferred it. Dr. Hinter asked the staff to present the results at the Medical Quality Committee meeting. The staff presented and their study was well received. In fact, a few of the other physicians have asked the nurses on their units to think about possible research studies.

Evaluation of Case Study 3

Using the tool provided by Wolf and colleagues,[2] this unit displays proactive behaviors in transformational leadership, exemplary professional practice, structural empowerment, and new knowledge and innovations.

EXHIBIT 4.8	MOVING FROM PROACTIVE TO HIGH-PERFORMING			
	Reactive	**Responsive**	**Proactive**	**High Performance**
Research	Research is not strongly valued.	Nurses may participate in research projects, but they rarely initiate research.	Nurses generate research and apply research to their practice.	Nurses are actively involved in generating and disseminating research on a national or international level.

Source: Wolf et al., 2014; reprinted with permission.

Reviewing the Case Study of a High-Performing Organization

If it appears that this organization is hard to believe, it is. High-performing units, organizations, and individuals are not easily found. Instead, aspects of high-performing people or units are found interspersed throughout an organization. High-performing organizations have a high level of synergy, innovation, and creativity. These organizations have the structures, processes, and outcomes to be recognized as a Magnet organization. The Preface page 1 of the *Magnet Manual* states, "ANCC's Magnet designation is the highest and most prestigious credential a healthcare organization can achieve for nursing excellence and quality patient care."[3] By reading the case study for high-performing organizations, one can see how the organization is a leader in all five components of the Magnet Model. These include Transformational Leadership; Structural Empowerment; Exemplary Professional Practice; New Knowledge, Innovations, and Improvements, and Empirical Outcomes.

One item to note in high-performing organizations is the way they lead. Nelson and Burns[1] describe the leadership style as holistic. Holistic leadership looks at how systems interconnect in order to continuously adapt, transform, and coordinate patient care delivery. Employees create learning environments, walk the talk, "dare to care," and focus on results.[7]

EXHIBIT
4.9

CASE STUDY 4: A HIGH-PERFORMING ORGANIZATION

Cooklebook Hospital just submitted an abstract for the ANCC National Magnet Conference® on innovative ideas for education. The abstract is not unusual for the organization; Cooklebook is frequently accepted to speak at the Magnet conference. Cooklebook was just recognized as one of the top 100 hospitals in the nation and has also been recognized by several other organizations for exceptional care.

Within the nursing division, more than 10 articles have been published in peer-reviewed journals. Cooklebook is currently involved in eight research studies, of which five are multidisciplinary. The CNO has been asked to speak at numerous hospitals about their Journey to Magnet Excellence® and sits on the board of the American Organization of Nurse Executives. Everyone on the leadership team is certified in a specialty and 60% of the nurses are certified. Over 80% of nurses at Cooklebook have a BSN; 20% of those also have a master's degree.

The latest report shows Cooklebook in the top decile for patient satisfaction. In the past two years, 70% of the units haven't had a fall with major injury, and less than 4% of patients have had a nosocomial infection in the past year. It is no surprise that Cooklebook has no vacancies and a waiting list of nurses wanting to work there. A nurse interviewed stated, "I have endless opportunities at Cooklebook. If you dream it, you can make it happen, here."

Evaluation of Case Study 4

Using the tool provided by Wolf and colleagues,[2] one can easily see how the organization in the case study is high performing.

	EXHIBIT 4.10	A HIGH-PERFORMING ORGANIZATION			

	Reactive	Responsive	Proactive	High Performance
Strategic Planning	Strategic planning is seen as a leadership responsibility and as a paper exercise with no tangible benefit nor involvement by staff nurses. There is limited alignment to individual or unit goals and activities.	The CNO solicits input from staff in designing the strategic plan, but nurses are not an integral part of the process. The primary focus is on short-term operational goals.	Nurses at all levels are involved in leveraging their clinical expertise in identifying ways to improve practice, which is reflected in the strategic plan. Nurses can articulate their contributions to the plan.	Nurses and nursing leadership use strategic planning to design their future vision, and can link the plan to tangible outcomes.

Source: Wolf et al., 2014; reprinted with permission.

CONCLUSION

Understanding the four developmental levels and being able to accurately assess progress of units, organizations, and individuals is a critical first step for leaders on the journey to excellence. Understanding these levels as applied to the Magnet Recognition Program® standards provides a framework for assessment and direction for achieving the next level.

The authors would like to gratefully acknowledge the contributions of Dr. Gail Wolf to this section.

REFERENCES

1. Nelson, L., & Burns, F. L. (1984). High performance programming: A framework for transforming organizations. In J. D. Adams (Ed.), *Transforming Work* (pp. 226–242). Alexandria, VA: Miles River Press.

2. Wolf, G., Finlayson, S., Hayden, M., Hoolahan, S., & Mazzoccoli, A. (2014). The developmental levels in achieving Magnet® designation, Part 1. *Journal of Nursing Administration, 44*(3), 136–141.

3. American Nurses Credentialing Center. (2019). *2019 Magnet Application Manual*. Silver Spring, MD: Author.

4. Kofter, J. P. (2007, January). Leading change: Why transformation efforts fail. *Harvard Business Review*, 92–107.

5. Hersey, P., & Blanchard, K. H. (1993*). Management of organizational behavior: Utilizing human resources (6th ed.).* Englewood Cliffs, NJ: Prentice-Hall.

6. Bass, B. M., Avolio, B. J., Jung, D. I., & Berson, Y. (2003). Predicting unit performance by assessing transformational and transactional leadership. *Journal of Applied Psychology*, *88*(2), 207.

7. Best, K. Candis (2011) Holistic leadership: A model for leader-member engagement and development. *Journal of Values-Based Leadership*, *4*(1); 5. Retrieved from http://scholar.valpo.edu/jvbl/vol4/iss1/5

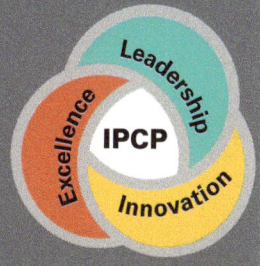

DESIGNING YOUR INNOVATION JOURNEY

STEP
5

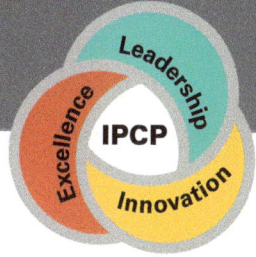

DESIGNING YOUR INNOVATION JOURNEY

It's important not to do the same old things in the same old way, but to push them to the limit and see what happens.

—Rod Judkins, *Pushing Your Envelope,* special *Time* edition

DESIGNING INNOVATION THAT WORKS

When you Google "innovation definition," you are presented with plethora of options. Likewise, when you try "innovation tools," "innovation models," or "innovation processes," you are returned hundreds of millions of choices. So where and how do you begin your innovation journey? How do you know what is the best innovation fit for your organization? This step reviews innovation fundamentals and is designed to help you explore innovation concepts and tools that will empower you to chart your organization's innovation strategies and tactics.

RECOMMENDED READING

Thomas, T. W., Seifert, P. C., & Joyner, J. C. (2016). Registered nurses leading innovative changes. *Online Journal of Issues in Nursing, 18*(3), manuscript 3.

Honan, L., Shealy, S., Fennie, K., Duffy, T. C., Friedlaender, L., & Del Vecchio, M. (2016). Looking Is Not Seeing and Listening Is Not Hearing: A Replication Study With Accelerated BSN Students, *Journal of Professional Nursing, 32*(Suppl. 5), S30–S36.

Everett, L. Q., & Sitterding, M. C. (2013). Building a culture of innovation by maximizing the role of the RN. *Nursing Administration Quarterly, 37*(3), 194–202.

WHAT IS INNOVATION?

Innovation is often described with a variety of terms and definitions, which frequently means that people are not talking about the same thing—they have personal ideas about innovation based on their experience. The concept of innovation dates back to the 1930s when Joseph Schumpeter, an economist, coined the definition as being a novel combination of knowledge, resources, and other factors to carry out commercialization of a new or newly combined idea.[1] Since Schumpeter's innovation theory, new constructs of innovation have emerged. Common features of innovation definitions relate to:

- Having a process in place to create something new using existing resources or combinations of new resources with old ones,

- Creating something that brings value to a target market, and

- Having a business model that delivers a return on investment for time and resources committed to implement an innovation.

The Global Innovation Index (GII) is an annual tracking report that started in 2007, with a goal to find metrics that accurately capture and measure global innovation in society. Collecting this data was deemed important because understanding innovation drivers is essential to gauge economic benefits of policies, competitive landscapes, and progress across nations. The 2019 GII report focuses on trends in healthcare and medical innovation,[2] linking GII measures to the global SDG 3 goal discussed in Step 1. "[The 2019] GII model includes 129 countries/economies, which represent 91.8% of the world's population and 96.8% of the world's GDP in purchasing power parity in current international dollars" (p. 206). The index includes 80 measures summarized into three primary measures—Innovation Input, Innovation Output, and an Overall GII country index score. Step 7: Tools and Resources presents an example of the 80 measures used to calculate the score using the U.S. trend analysis report. The GII framework reflects a broad perspective of drivers that impact innovation.

GII's definition of innovation is based on international standards that have been updated with *Oslo Manual 2018: Guidelines for Collecting, Reporting and Using Data on Innovation, 4th Edition,* prepared by OECD/Eurostat. The manual focuses on business activities required to conduct innovation and how to measure activities over time. It provides support to identify adjustments needed to capture innovation process measures for differences in business activities (e.g., type of firm), type of innovation being pursued (incremental or disruptive for product or process innovations), and other factors needed to customize innovation measures to specific requirements of an organization. The Oslo Manual's high-level definition of innovation is as follows:

> **An innovation is a new or improved product or process (or combination thereof) that differs significantly from the unit's previous products or processes and that has been made available to potential users (product) or brought into use by the unit (process).**

Source: 2018 Oslo Manual, p. 20[3]

The GII framework looks at five enabling **innovation inputs**: Institutions, Human Capital and Research, Infrastructure, Market Sophistication, and Business Sophistication. Innovation progress is reflected in measured **innovation outputs**: Knowledge and Technology, and Creative Outputs. The result is the assignment of a **GII country index score** that combines input and output index scores.

The GII report highlights the complexity of gauging innovation across organizations and nations. The study authors do not portend to claim that the GII country index scores are the ultimate or only innovation measures to be considered. Instead, they present a case that many factors need to be studied, and factor selection influences innovation model designs, measures and outputs, and reporting of results.

Given the diversity and complexity of innovation data, it is realistic that innovation takes on unique meanings and perceptions about what it is and what it is not. Exercise 5.1 can help broaden your thinking about factors to consider as you select your innovation model and design your innovation process.

As you explore different innovation models to support your organization, you will need to declare:

- What you mean by innovation,
- What factors you will consider as inputs and outputs,
- How you will track results to improve organizational progress, and
- How you will gauge your progress relative to your internal goals and competitors.

Reflection Exercise

Using the GII country rankings, consider how you can introduce innovation models to your organization.

The 2019 GII report offers a perspective on the breadth of factors needed to capture global innovation progress. Use the GII country scores to highlight the various factors included in the GII country index score. A discussion about the variety of measures included, measure consistency required to ensure quality comparisons, and issues encountered to collect data should be examined.

Exemplar: GII Country Rankings Can Impact Innovation Strategies and Tactics

According to the 2019 GII rankings, for the ninth consecutive year Switzerland ranked as the world leader in innovation. Comparatively, the United States moved up to the third position worldwide and improved input and output index scores in five of the seven categories. It ranked first in Market Sophistication (credit, investment, trade, competition, and market scale) and second in Business Sophistication (knowledge workers, innovation linkages, and knowledge absorption). In quality of innovation measures, the United States ranked first with quality of universities contributing to its place in global rankings. (For ranking details by country, the full report can be accessed at https://www.wipo.int/edocs/pubdocs/en/wipo_pub_gii_2019.pdf.)

Health care is experiencing significant disruptions brought forth by new competitors, funding modifications, regulatory and healthcare worker licensure changes, and technological revolutions such as artificial intelligence and big data. The 2019 GII report estimates that $177 billion will be invested worldwide on healthcare innovation activities, with medical technology patents significantly driving investment growth. According to the WIPO Statistics database, for the period 2010–2017 the United States led the number of patent

2019 Country Rankings[4]

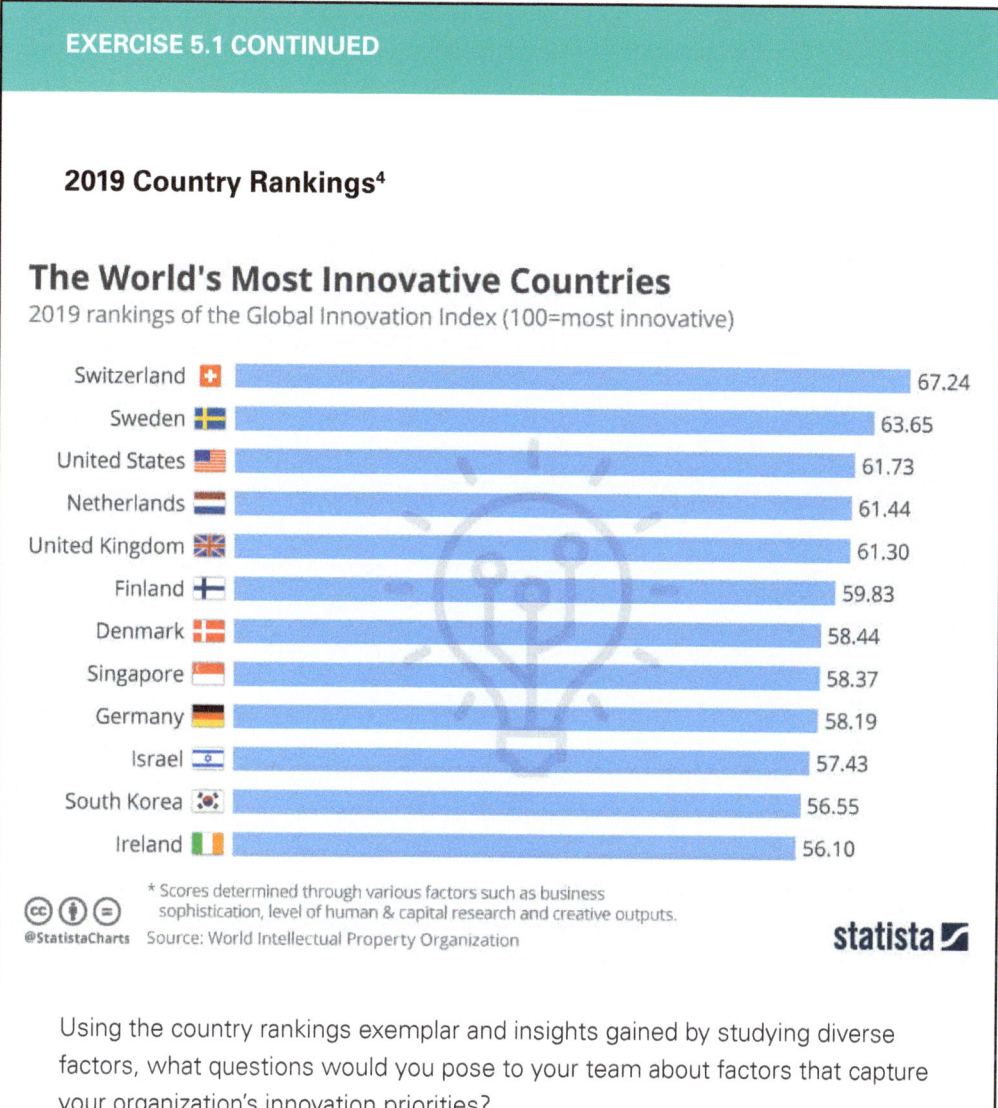

The World's Most Innovative Countries
2019 rankings of the Global Innovation Index (100=most innovative)

Switzerland	67.24
Sweden	63.65
United States	61.73
Netherlands	61.44
United Kingdom	61.30
Finland	59.83
Denmark	58.44
Singapore	58.37
Germany	58.19
Israel	57.43
South Korea	56.55
Ireland	56.10

* Scores determined through various factors such as business sophistication, level of human & capital research and creative outputs.

@StatistaCharts   Source: World Intellectual Property Organization

statista

Using the country rankings exemplar and insights gained by studying diverse factors, what questions would you pose to your team about factors that capture your organization's innovation priorities?

publications worldwide in medical technology (284,223) and biotechnology (126,581), and placed second in pharmaceutical patents (204,057). China led in pharmaceutical patents (214,992) during this same period[2] (p. 48).

The GII report identified five drivers of global healthcare innovation[5] (pp. 87–88):

- **Information Revolution**: broadband access, new smartphone and other IoT (Internet of Things) devices, data such as genomic information, and use of electronic health records that store structured and unstructured data.

- **Artificial Intelligence**: data access coupled with affordable and efficient computing and storage. New applications will augment healthcare practitioners and will supplement global areas with new healthcare applications that address local healthcare worker shortages.

- **Targeted Treatments**: custom products for personalized, targeted therapies based on new science, biomarker advances, and the development of niche medicines.

- **Consumerism:** Consumers are paying for more healthcare expenses and are incentivized to pursue alternative treatments and providers of care. As out-of-pocket (OOP) costs increase, expectations regarding customer service and the availability and quality of care will continue to rise.

- **Business Model Changes**: New payment and provider models are breaking down traditional silos of providers, payers, insurers, and employers. Public-private partnerships are evolving.

The GII report also captures predictions regarding innovation priorities that will drive future global innovations. Exhibit 5.1 presents the report's findings. Today, investments are following the priority categories. While no one can predict the future, it is likely that we will continue to see significant growth in these areas of healthcare innovation.

INNOVATION IS TODAY'S GOLD RUSH

In 2000, innovation experts Christensen and colleagues predicted that "the great growth opportunities exist in the simpler tiers of the market."[6] In 2014, $6.5 billion was invested in new healthcare start-ups, with significant investments going toward big data analytics and population health management, patient engagement, and personalized medicine.[7] Then, 2015 saw an explosion of healthcare solutions aimed toward consumer mass markets as well as artificial intelligence and big data applications.

Dreamit Ventures estimated that in Q1 2018, $1.62 billion was invested in digital health start-ups.[8] Based on a data analysis prepared by Pitchbook, a venture capital–tracking research firm, by the end of Q4 2018, *Forbes* estimated that $28.8 billion would be raised for healthcare deals.[9]

Today, healthcare consumers have access to simple inventions such as digital pill boxes that monitor compliance, smartphones that can track their vital signs while engaging them in medical research, nurse–patient care coordination tools to help monitor healthcare progress, remote telemedicine accessible through web applications, and access to a wide

EXHIBIT 5.1   INNOVATIONS DRIVING THE FUTURE OF HEALTH CARE

Promising fields for medical innovation and technologies

NEW SCIENTIFIC BREAKTHROUGHS TREATMENTS, AND CURES

Genetics and stem cell research
— Single-cell analysis
— Gene and stem cell therapies
— Gene engineering and editing including CRISPR technology

Nanotechnology
— Swallowable small devices

Biologics
— Development and manufacture of complex biologics

Brain research, neurology, and neurosurgery
— Characterization of the brain's major circuits
— New brain imagery for mental disorders
— Migraine treatment

New generation of vaccines and immunotherapy
— HIV and universal flu vaccine
— Cancer vaccine
— Immunotherapy
— New vaccine delivery methods

Pain management
— Effective, non-addictive medicines for pain management

Mental health treatments
— Pre-symptomatic diagnosis and treatment of Alzheimer's disease and other cognitive declines

NEW MEDICAL TECHNOLOGIES

Medical devices
— 3D printing
— Cardiac devices
— Implants and bionics

Medical imaging and diagnostics
— Optical high-definition imaging and virtual anatomic models
— Biosensors and markers
— 4D human charting and virtual reality
— Screening for diseases

Precision and personalized medicine
— Computer-assisted surgery
— Surgical robots
— Personalized medicine

Regenerative medicine
— Tissue engineering
— Effective bioartificial pancreas

ORGANIZATIONAL AND PROCESS INNOVATIONS

Novel approaches in healthcare research
— Software-based modeling to speed up research
— Artificial intelligence techniques to speed up research and clinical trials

New ways of delivering healthcare
— Telemedicine applications
— Drone delivery of medications
— Remote monitoring and portable diagnostics
— Improved data sharing

Sources: GII 2019 chapters, in particular Collins, 2010. Also Kraft, 2019, Nature 2018, Nature 2019, Frost & Sullivan 2018, Frost & Sullivan 2019, European Commission 2007, Medical Futurist 2017, Mesko 2018.

Cornell University, INSEAD, and WIPO (2019); The Global Innovation Index 2019: Creating Healthy Lives-The Future of Medical Innovation, Ithaca, Fountainbleau, and Geneva. Used with permission.

variety of medical applications that travel with them on their smartphones and tablets.[10–12] The Deloitte Center for Health Solutions claims that digital healthcare transformation is the result of a convergence of four significant trends: the availability of new technologies, consumers' increasing demand for healthcare value, expanding healthcare consumption rates, and government influences.[13] These factors are supported by other research sources and should be evaluated for effects on your organization when you conduct your environmental scan of competitive marketplace conditions.

With no end in sight to investments in health care we need to ask, "Will innovations contribute to our rising healthcare costs or will they help bend the cost curve?"

WHY HEALTHCARE INNOVATION MATTERS

In the United States, primary drivers of innovation in health care are about achieving the National Quality Strategy (NQS) aims for better care, healthy people/healthy communities, and affordable care, and having the ability to respond to emerging healthcare opportunities as new technologies, processes, and changing consumer demands unfold. The passage of the Affordable Care Act in 2010 included the creation of the NQS to guide a nationwide quality effort, and the development of a Center for Medicare & Medicaid Innovation (CMMI) to test "innovative program and service delivery models to reduce program expenditures . . . while preserving or enhancing the quality of care" for people who receive Medicare, Medicaid, or Children's Health Insurance Program (CHIP) benefits.[14] Key drivers for the creation of the CMMI were projected growth rates in program costs[15] and quality-of-care concerns[16] related to patient-level outcomes and patient-centered criteria. In 2010, the CMMI was provided a total of $10 billion to fund 2011–2019 innovation projects. As of November 2018, there were 41 delivery models being tested (see https://innovation.cms.gov/initiatives /#views=models).

By 2027, it is estimated that U.S. healthcare expenditures will reach $6 trillion, representing 19.4% of the GDP. The Peterson-Kaiser Health System Tracker provides perspective. By 2027, healthcare spending in the United States will reach $16,907 for each and every man, woman, and child .[17] For our healthcare investments, do we receive better access, quality, and outcomes as compared to other nations? According to the Commonwealth Fund healthcare data, the answer is no (see https://www.commonwealthfund.org/health-system -performance-and-costs). The United States spends more than any other comparable developed nation yet experiences wide variations in access, quality, and outcomes. Given the magnitude of the problem and the potential return on investment for innovations, it is not surprising that new competitors armed with money and resources are flowing into this sector. Exhibit 5.2 from the Health System Tracker shows what a –1% swing from baseline healthcare cost projections would yield if we could bend the cost curve on our national healthcare expenditures.

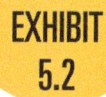

EXHIBIT 5.2

HEALTHCARE SPENDING PROJECTIONS

Projected annual change in U.S. per capita health spending 2018– 2027, alternative scenarios

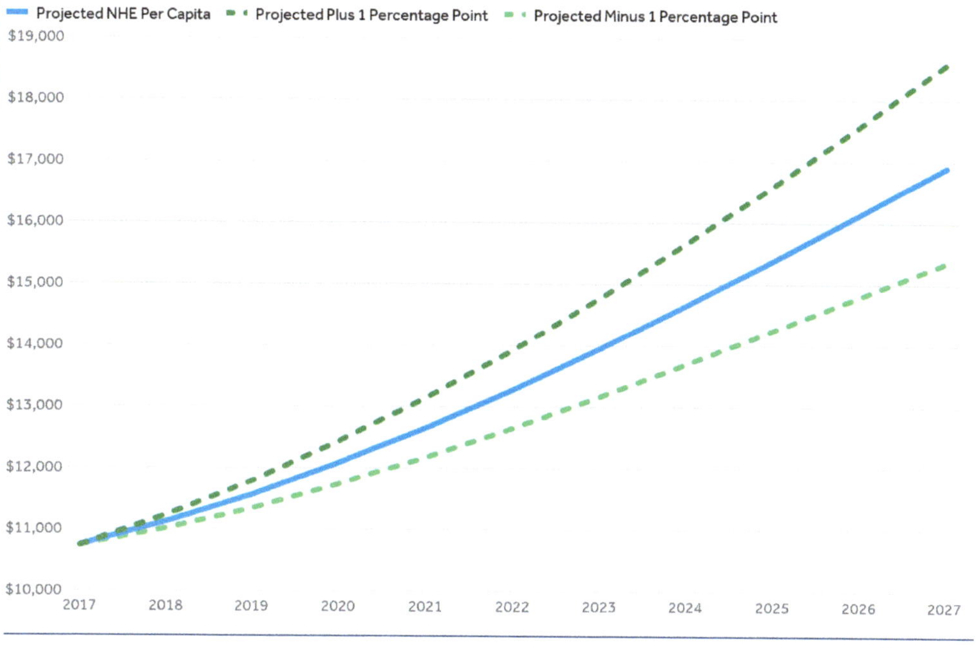

— Projected NHE Per Capita   ▪ ▪ Projected Plus 1 Percentage Point   ▪ ▪ Projected Minus 1 Percentage Point

Source: KFF analysis of National Health Expenditure Accounts (NHEA) • Get the data • PNG

Peterson-Kaiser
Health System Tracker

Kamal, R., Sawyer, B., McDermott, D. & Kaiser Family Foundation. *How much is health spending expected to grow?*, (Peterson-Kaiser Health System Tracker, [March 12, 2019])

A report by the BCG Henderson Institute supports Exhibit 5.2 projections. The BCG research found "wide variations in health outcomes across hospitals, regions, and countries, with no clear causal relationship between money invested and health delivered. . . . There is growing evidence that a substantial portion of healthcare spending is, quite simply, wasted on avoidable medical complications or on medically unnecessary treatments."[18]

New competitors in the healthcare industry are turning common business models upside down. Google entered the healthcare market with Google Glass in 2013, and while there was much enthusiasm about the potential of the device, no one really understood how it would change health care—although enthusiastic consumer and business explorers competed to pay $1,500 to experience the first release of the product.[19] Fast-forward to 2019 and we find that Google has redesigned features and applications for the device, changing its target market to enterprise applications versus the initial consumer-focused market.[20]

Also take notice of what Google did when it reorganized the company as Alphabet. Google created Verily, a company focused on healthcare data analytics. Not losing sight of the potential to cross-pollinate products and services, Google teams formed projects that crossed Google companies such as Deep Mind, Google's artificial intelligence research lab. In 2013 Google also launched Calico, a company focused on health and well-being that seeks to research and tackle aging. Google is into health care for the long haul.[21]

Not to be left behind, Apple entered the health market with health applications available on your watch and iPhone. Apple targets both consumers and healthcare organizations with a mix of healthcare applications, seeking to transform the healthcare "practitioner-patient" relationship with new tools and ways of working together to improve healthcare outcomes. In 2018, Apple obtained FDA clearance letters for its EKG and irregular rhythm notifications on its Apple Watch Series 4 product.[22] To gain access to enterprise markets, Apple now works with start-ups to develop applications that can change healthcare delivery.

Tired of rising healthcare costs, in 2018 Amazon, Berkshire Hathaway, and JPMorgan Chase & Company formed a joint healthcare company called Haven. The company is charged with finding ways to transform healthcare and to provide their employees primary care access with simplified insurance benefits at more affordable prices. The three organizations employ 1.2 million workers and family members, and Haven is deemed a viable competitor to established insurance and healthcare providers.[23]

Telehealth is a market of innovation unto itself. It has been around for over a decade but is now being recognized as a viable solution to save billions on healthcare expenditures.[24] While the utilization of telehealth as an option has been mixed, as technology and digital access improve, it is predicted that consumers will begin to embrace this approach to healthcare delivery. A primary reason for predicted consumer adoption is convenience and cost. Adoption of the technology requires a restructuring of healthcare delivery regulations across state lines, and the transformation of practitioner processes to integrate telehealth care delivery models into daily practice.[25]

Seeing an opportunity in the pharmacy sector to deliver prescriptions to consumers, in 2018 Amazon purchased PillPack, a company that delivers medications in white packets labeled with prescription information and schedules for administration, making it easier for people to remember when and how to take prescriptions. Looking to its consumer market, Amazon sees the $500 billion prescription drug market as an opportunity to better serve existing Amazon customers and to potentially gain new ones.[26] The acquisition has the capability to upend the pharmacy industry.

The new disruptors facing off with existing players in traditional markets should encourage organizations to, at a minimum, annually assess trending market dynamics and partnerships—acquisitions, mergers, and new innovators are rapidly entering the $3.5+ trillion healthcare market. The influx of billions of dollars into the redesign or creation of products and services is certain to change the face of healthcare delivery. Selecting how you will innovate and establish supporting infrastructures, whom you potentially will partner with, and how much to invest in transforming your organization are critical strategic decisions.

Based on his experience in transforming organizations and investing in future technologies, Dr. James L. Madara, CEO and executive vice president of the American Medical Association (AMA), offers insight about what to consider when establishing innovation investments and how to partner with others to accomplish audacious innovations.

ADVICE ON HOW TO SHOOT FOR THE MOON

Establishing a thriving innovation ecosystem is hard work and requires patience. Pause and reorientation are sometimes necessary, and mindset can be more important than footprint.

—Dr. James Madara

In 2016, the AMA became a founding partner of Health2047, a Silicon Valley start-up focused on developing new products, tools, and resources to improve the practice of medicine and the delivery of care. AMA describes its investment as an opportunity to combine physician expertise with technology advancements that can transform a $3+ trillion healthcare industry. AMA explains itself as redefining how 21st-century associations can operate by actively participating in creating solutions that address health-sector challenges. Dr. Madara describes the Health2047 mission as taking on "moonshot-level challenges that require audacious effort and uncompromising commitment." He offers advice on how to achieve success when shooting for the moon.[27]

EXHIBIT 5.3 **SIX INVESTMENT PRINCIPLES FOR AUDACIOUS INNOVATION**

1. Focus on the North Star

The AMA's mission is to promote the art and science of medicine and the betterment of public health, our North Star. When calibrating strategic investment, this North Star creates a double bottom line. We can generate terrific financial returns on AMA-backed innovation ventures, but this alone does not meet our success criteria. Our investments must also supply improvement in approaches to chronic disease, health data organization and flow, physician productivity, and value. A typical investor may seek a 3x financial return to compensate for the risk premium. The terms are purely financial. But our double bottom line is drawn under the AMA North Star, so advancing our mission also weighs greatly in measuring return on investment.

EXHIBIT 5.3 CONTINUED

2. Touchdowns, not field goals

The demands of principle #1 dictate that any supported venture will be both pre-competitive and transformative by nature. There are worthy health technology ventures that are connected, evidence-based, clinically validated, and critical to some specialization of medicine. But these attributes alone do not satisfy our rules—they aren't aiming high enough. To warrant inclusion in our innovation ecosystem, ventures must demonstrate broadly transformational impact.

3. Saving lives takes more time than developing theories on how to do so

Our perspective is devoted to enabling practical application and we know it's a long game. Consider that, after launch, it takes 12 years on average for a biomedical startup to exit. Or consider that we're currently facing 35 years of market-driven applications focused on administrative needs (a market that comprises $3.5 trillion/18% of GDP). This has to be corrected and we feel the urgency, but urgency must be tempered with innovations that are evidence based, validated, and actionable.

4. Pursuit of the perfect is the enemy of the good

Variations of this concept have been attributed to Voltaire, Confucius, and Shakespeare. If we follow our North Star, make touchdowns, and do more than we theorize, we can initially shape the direction of ventures, iteratively move along, and attract other investments. But as these ventures mature, our influence will become diluted. To have an important role in a larger ecosystem—comprised of interconnected players with specific roles of contribution and consumption—we must be a real part of that ecosystem, and that means we won't always be 100% in control of our investments. We are in the space of good; let's not think it has to be perfect.

5. Fuel is fuel

We can't 100% control what happens years after our backed ventures launch and companies develop through additional rounds of investment. But we can very much bias them toward our North Star by the act of creation and early guidance—and later partnership. Consider how the AMA generates revenue and income: Its "fuel" comes from a combination of membership, products, digital content, and publishing. We appreciate these many revenue streams that allow us to accomplish our mission. Likewise, if Health2047 ventures benefit from AMA operating funds, seed support, capital partners investment, customer capital infusion, IP licensing . . . it's all good. Fuel is fuel and variation is healthy.

6.   Turn the pathetic into the enviable

Just as the USSR's Sputnik triumph in 1957 launched the space race and the magnificence of NASA, the dismal state of healthcare technology can be turned to advantage. Medicine lags far behind in using tech advances now common in parallel industries (our data problems alone are pitiable). But this pathetic state can be made enviable, as we apply others' hard-won approaches, developed over decades, to remedy our lag. Much of the technology sector and its R&D dollars are focused on creating the next big thing. The healthcare industry can strategically take the best existing technology (already developed, tested, proven, and refined)—and judiciously apply it to modernizing medicine following principles #1–5!

Source: Dr. James L. Madara, 2019. AMA © 2019. Used with permission.

SETTING INNOVATION TARGETS

Innovation efforts can be well-designed incremental enhancements to existing services or processes, or they can be initiatives that are completely novel, leading to significant disruptions in the marketplace. Given the high stakes, time commitments, failure rates, and high cost of pursuing disruptive innovations, most innovations focus on incremental efforts. Exhibit 5.4 provides examples of incremental and disruptive innovations.

The Robert Wood Johnson (RWJ) Foundation's bold initiative, *Creating a Culture of Health: Pioneering Ideas*, targets innovations that inspire fresh thinking and solutions that can be applied to "spark a continual exchange of ideas that could help us all live healthier, happier and longer."[31] The RWJ website (http://www.rwjf.org/en/how-we-work/grants/what-we-fund /submit-a-proposal.html#checklist) provides an exemplar that lists essential business case information to assess innovation ideas (see Exhibit 5.5).

Nursing, in collaboration with interprofessional teams, must be positioned to implement processes and outcome-tracking capabilities that rapidly respond to changing healthcare environments.[32] With the passage of the 2010 Patient Protection and Affordable Care Act (ACA), a plethora of new innovation approaches and organizations supporting experimentation have emerged. Because there is not a "one size fits all" approach to innovation, each organization must carefully assess its own culture, processes, and available resources to execute innovation projects that can yield a return on investment or advance the field of

EXHIBIT
5.4

EXAMPLES OF INCREMENTAL AND DISRUPTIVE INNOVATION

Innovation efforts need to address a specific problem, an identified market gap or an opportunity to take advantage of emerging trends ahead of competitors.

—Nancy Robert, PhD, MBA, BSN–Managing Partner, Polaris Solutions

Incremental: The use of digital fitness tracking devices rapidly became mainstream (it is estimated that 75% of adults now use a fitness tracker[28]) with improvements now focused on collecting more data and integrating data with other sources of information. This is incremental innovation—ideas that build on existing products or processes that can be recombined or enhanced in new and exciting ways.

Disruptive: Google launched Google Glass, a hands-free computerized eyeglass technology deemed transformative by technology pundits and beta-test customers. The product was envisioned as a new device that could link advanced analytics capabilities, such as IBM's artificial intelligence Watson engine, with the user experience. The healthcare industry was a key target market, and incubators such as Glassomics® were formed to test out the new user interface paradigm.[19] The initial product launch failed—often an outcome of daring undertakings.

Google placed a big bet on the new technology, and like many first-time disruptive innovation attempts, it failed. In January 2015 Google pulled the product from the market, stating that "[it] had broken ground and allowed us to learn what's important to consumers and enterprises alike . . . we will work to integrate those learnings into future products."[29] Fast-forward to July and the market had multiple next-generation eyeglass competitors.

The initial idea was a novel technology paradigm that attracted new entrants into a potential market opportunity. This is an example of a disruptive innovation: it's a potential game-changer.

Tenacity prevailed, and in 2017 a new Google Glass product emerged and is now driving applications and new workflows within multiple industries.[30]

EXHIBIT 5.5

IDENTIFYING SUSTAINABLE INNOVATIONS

To help you evaluate how your innovation idea compares with other innovations, consider:

Novelty — Is this something that is completely new, or is this an improvement on prior products or processes?

Progressive — How does your idea break away from traditional thinking? How will others view your idea? Does the environmental scan support progressive thinking?

Transformational — Does the idea radically challenge the status quo? What will it take to recruit ambassadors to support the idea to get it into practice?

Interdisciplinary — Does your project propose to bring in perspectives from other industries or draw together uncommon partners? Are you prepared to manage the relationships?

Potential Impact — Does your idea address a large-scale problem in terms of finances, resources, geographic differences, or other impact factors to be considered? Is the idea specific to addressing one problem or can it be applied to other domains?

Viability — Does your idea have the potential to produce outcomes that would be valued and that would engage others to replicate the idea?

health care. As the Deloitte Center for Health Solutions points out, "Innovations have to 'earn their keep.'"[13]

Successful innovations begin with sorting through which projects may be the most valuable investments of time, resources, and organizational commitments. Exhibit 5.6 details questions you should consider when starting an innovation project.

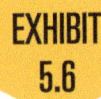

EXHIBIT 5.6

INNOVATION PROJECT CRITERIA

Innovation Plan Considerations

Define the Process

We know an organization needs a well-defined process to successfully innovate, yet the Product Development Institute's research suggests that over 60% of U.S.-based companies do not have an innovation strategy. You can create a winning plan if you:

- Declare what you are trying to achieve by creating a portfolio of innovation projects. Why are you asking others to invest time and resources and risk failure?

- Make sure your innovation model integrates with your strategic planning process at all levels of the organization.

- Declare your innovation intentions and do not assume that once stated, all is understood. Launch a campaign to engage the organization in the innovation process and repeat as needed.

- Clearly define what is and is not included in each step of your model and define how milestones and progress will be measured.

- Identify how ideas will be generated, collected, sorted, and evaluated, with results communicated (go and no-go decisions).

- Train innovation project team members using well-documented innovation terms and conditions of participation. Training and explaining are the first steps to engaging the organization in a cultural transformation aimed toward embracing an innovation process.

Establish Clear Project Decision Criteria

- How do you select and fund innovation projects in your organization?

- If an innovation project is pursued, will funds be reduced in other departments? Is there a special fund that allows teams to risk resources and potentially fail?

- What project decision criteria will be used? Decision criteria need to be explicit, consistent, and clearly communicated within the organization. Criteria used to sort through initial ideas will differ from criteria used to sort pilot project results.

EXHIBIT 5.6 CONTINUED

Everyone in the organization needs to be informed about selection criteria, and they must believe that the criteria are applied fairly—no special considerations. Special pet projects are innovation-killers.

Identify the Problem or Opportunity Being Pursued

- What problem are you trying to solve?
- What opportunity are you trying to pursue?
- What evidence suggests the problem or opportunity exists?
- Do others in the organization view this problem or opportunity as being significant or relevant to clinical or operational success?
- Does the problem or opportunity affect current strategic plans?
- On a scale of 1 to 5 (1 not critical to 5 extremely critical), how would you rate the importance of this problem or opportunity?
- Is there an executive sponsor willing to commit time and resources to this problem or opportunity?
- Given the organizational culture, is it possible to pursue this problem or opportunity?

Establish Targeted Outcomes (ROI, clinical, or operational)

- What is the expected outcome if the project is pursued?
- How difficult will it be to measure the outcome?
- To what degree does the outcome matter?
- Who in the organization will be affected by the outcome? Do they agree that the problem or opportunity should be pursued?

IDENTIFYING AN INNOVATION MODEL THAT IS RIGHT FOR YOUR ORGANIZATION

While many models of innovation are in use today, models typically share common features based on findings from innovation research, experience (successes and failures), and dissemination capabilities within organizations. At its core, innovation is:

- A defined process;

- Designed to address a specific problem, challenge, or opportunity; and

- Aimed to achieve a targeted outcome that is valued.

According to Danielle Cass, an innovation evangelist for Kaiser Permanente, by connecting people we can best cross-pollinate ideas, share learning, celebrate successes, and generate enthusiasm for new ways of thinking—ultimately leading to improvements in the quality of care or services provided to patients and communities.[33] Pisano in the *Harvard Business Review* points out that to be successful you need to be armed with a well-articulated innovation strategy that establishes "a set of coherent, mutually reinforcing policies or behaviors aimed at achieving a specific competitive goal."[34] An innovation plan provides a structure to align strategic and business priorities, to establish networks of people who are mutually supportive and interested in innovation projects, and affords opportunities to identify and disseminate best practices within an organization.

Each organization must determine its tolerance level for innovation and its capabilities to execute innovation projects. Given the abundance of innovation approaches available, it is critical that you gain detailed insights about your organizational environment before selecting an innovation model. Remember, there is no perfect model; the right model is the one that allows you to shape innovation processes according to your organizational needs.

Essential leadership traits to successfully execute and sustain an innovation model require different management thinking. Gone are the days of command and control; this has been replaced with a facilitation or coaching role required of innovation leaders. Leaders must have the capacity to think strategically while leading tactically, balance risk and reward of providing resources, be tenacious in the face of adversity, be supportive of ideation and creativity processes that encourage exploration while tracking evidence-based progress, embrace the unexpected and thrive in ambiguous conditions, and manage teams to achieve project timelines.[35–37]

EXHIBIT
5.7

CULTURE AND PROCESSES VITAL TO INNOVATION

While processes may differ in each organization, certain essential leadership traits are necessary to promote innovation activities and behaviors.

To accomplish anything, *transparency* is critical. Without it, you undermine organizational motivation to participate in any innovation process.

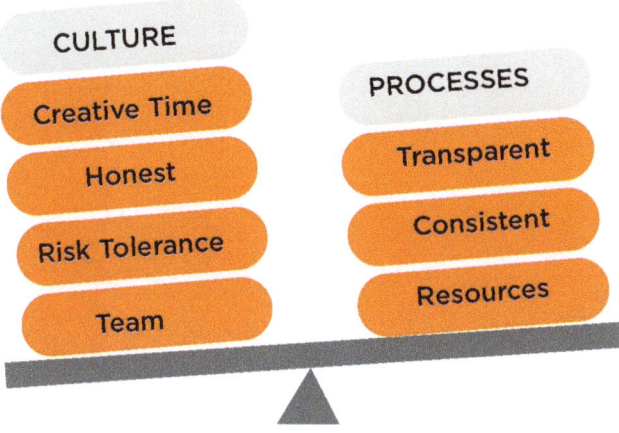

TEAM MATTERS

Teams make or break innovation efforts. While culture lays the foundation from which teams operate, team dynamics drive performance. In their groundbreaking work on extraordinary teams, Bellman and Ryan found eight indicators that are essential to achieving team outcomes.[38] As you review the team indicators, consider how you would rate teams within your organization. Note what you do well and areas that could improve (see Table 5.1).

TABLE 5.1
EIGHT INDICATORS OF EXTRAORDINARY TEAMS

INDICATOR	INDICATOR DESCRIPTION	RATING OF TEAM INTENT AND BEHAVIOR*
1. Compelling Purpose	Inspires members, stretching them as they make the group's work the priority	Rating:
2. Shared Leadership	Demonstrates members' mutual responsibility for initiating toward group success	Rating:
3. Just-Enough-Structure	Moves the group forward together without becoming fixed or burdensome	Rating:
4. Full Engagement	Shows in everyone's readiness to dive in with focus, enthusiasm, and passion—often chaotically	Rating:
5. Embracing of Differences	Results in a widened group perspective, creativity, and more options for action	Rating:
6. Unexpected Learning	Learning goes beyond the immediate task and is useful in other groups and life	Rating:
7. Strengthened Relationships	Shown in trust, interdependence, and friendships within the group	Rating:
8. Great Results	Including tangible outcomes organizations value and the intangible outcomes treasured by group members	Rating:

* 5 = Almost always fits, 4 = Fits much of the time, 3 = Fits about half the time, 2 = Occasionally fits, 1 = Seldom fits with my team

Source: Bellman & Ryan (2009). From *Extraordinary Groups: How Ordinary Teams Achieve Amazing Results*. Used with permission.

INNOVATION PROJECTS SHOULD SUPPORT STRATEGIC AND TACTICAL GOALS

Innovation projects and priorities should directly map to your organization's strategic plans and tactical goals, providing clarity regarding:

- What type of innovation you are pursuing: incremental or disruptive?

- How the innovation supports strategies and tactics identified in organizational plans.

- How the innovation supports changes in interprofessional practices, departmental roles and processes, and healthcare delivery—most importantly, does the innovation improve patient-centered care?

- What technology, space, and process advancements will be achieved if resources are committed to the innovation?

To get started, a small team should be convened to collect external environmental data that can be used to identify innovation priorities and critical linkages to your organization's strategic plans. External scans can provide insight into emerging trends and can help you anticipate potential challenges (see Exhibit 5.8).

EXHIBIT
5.8

CREATING AN ENVIRONMENTAL ANALYSIS

A great foundation to any strategic planning and innovation endeavor is to conduct an environmental scan and to identify the external factors that affect the way your organization operates. One useful tool for doing this is the PESTLE model, which is a mnemonic that stands for Political, Economic, Social, Technological, Legal, and Environmental. Created by Harvard professor Francis Aguilar in 1967, this model can be used alone or in combination with other tools to determine an organization's overall outlook. PESTLE is most often used when launching a new product or exploring a new market.

By making use of this tool, you can help ensure that your organization is aligned with its environment and avoid taking actions that are doomed to failure because of external factors. The primary purpose of the tool is to help you to identify as many relevant external factors as possible that may have an impact on your organization.

How to Use the Pestle Tool

- Brainstorm and list issues within each category.

- Identify the implications of each issue.

  - Consider relative importance to the organization.
  - Consider the likelihood of it occurring.

- Draw conclusions from this information.

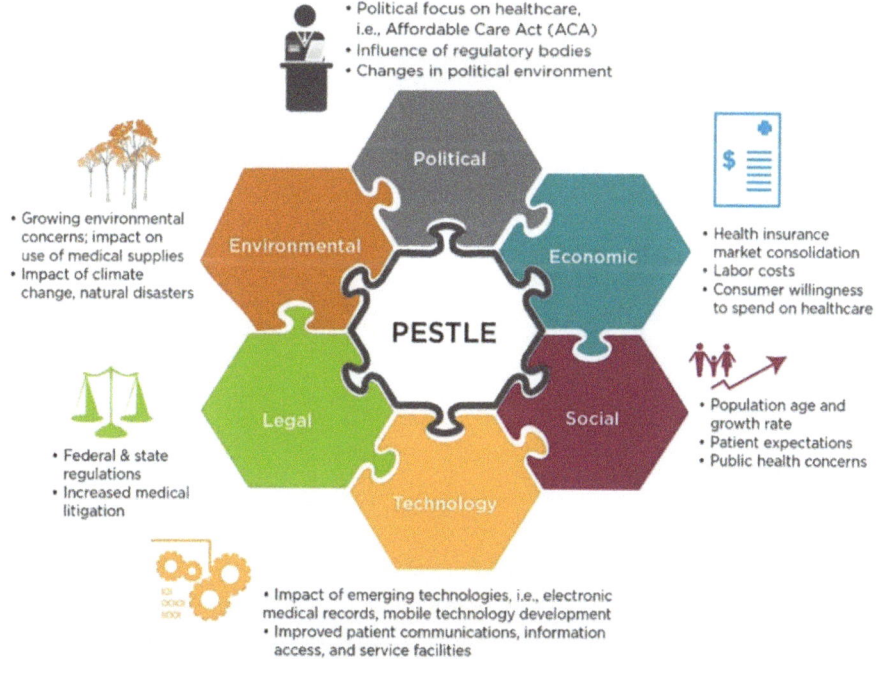

Once you are clear about strategic priorities, how do you align your thinking to embrace new possibilities? In *Step 7: Tools and Resources*, you will find Innovator Worksheets that can help your team navigate brainstorming opportunities while avoiding commonly known thinking pitfalls.

EXERCISE 5.2 — PESTLE PRACTICE WITH INTERPROFESSIONAL COLLABORATIVE TEAMS

- Form a group with about six team members. The team should have inter-professional participation.

- Download Deloitte's article, "The Convergence of Health Care Trends: Innovation Strategies for Emerging Opportunities," from http://www2. deloitte.com/us/en/pages/life-sciences-and-health-care/articles/ convergence-health-care-trends.html.

- Pair up in twos; each team should select one of the four significant trends in Deloitte's Figure 2 diagram on page 4 of the downloaded report. With your partner, move through the PESTLE wheel and write down your answers and any new questions you generate based on your discussion.

- Share your results with the group. Note similarities and differences in responses from each team. As the team works together, be careful that interprofessional team barriers do not impede your progress. Look for:

  - Equality among all team members—hierarchical thinking and lack of knowledge about roles can hamper acceptance of team member contributions.

  - Assess how the team works together using the Bellman-Ryan criteria (Table 5.1)— keep team dynamics on track.

COLLECTING RESULTS TO TRACK AND COMMUNICATE YOUR INNOVATION STORY

Whether you pursue incremental or disruptive innovations, of utmost importance is understanding and consistently applying how you will collect and measure the impact of your projects.

Innovation models capture some form of data to evaluate progress. ANCC's Magnet Recognition Program®, a program that defines standards of nursing excellence, demonstrates how linkages are established between innovation standards and measures. The Magnet Model requires empirical evidence of support for innovations that foster nursing research and dissemination of the research (standards NK1 & NK2*), use of evidence-based practices to improve nursing (standards NK3 & NK4), contributions to innovations in the organization (standard NK5), nurses' involvement with the design and launch of technology solutions to improve patient experiences and nursing practice (standard NK6EO), and engagement of nurses in work flow and space designs that lead to improvements that enhance nursing practice (standard NK7EO).[39] As you consider how to evaluate your ideas, design projects, and track your implementation outcomes, keep focused on what data you are going to monitor, how you will collect them, and how you will present your findings.

A useful resource to help you understand how data are connected to patient care quality measures is ANA's publication *Data Makes the Difference: The Smart Nurse's Handbook for Using Data to Improve Care*.[40] The book explains nursing quality and safety programs, and details data that you most likely will encounter as you link your nursing innovation strategy with the organization's strategic and tactical plans.

The pursuit of innovation is hard and complex, and typically requires the flexibility to pivot down uncharted paths. This makes it essential that you set up processes that allow you to know where you are headed (expected outcomes), readily respond to needed changes based on results (change management), and track where you have been (lessons learned).

A variety of tools can be used to set up and track your project outcomes. An example of a project tracking tool can be found at the Institute for Healthcare Improvement's (IHI) website.[41] The Multi-Tracking Tool is part of a toolkit prepared by Institute for Healthcare Improvement. The workbook can be accessed at http://www.ihi.org/resources/Pages/Tools/InnovationQuality ProjectSummarySheetMultiProjectTrackingTool.aspx. The tool highlights information needed to successfully manage an innovation project. Regardless of what tools you use to manage your progress, basic information such as that listed in Exhibit 5.9 will be required.

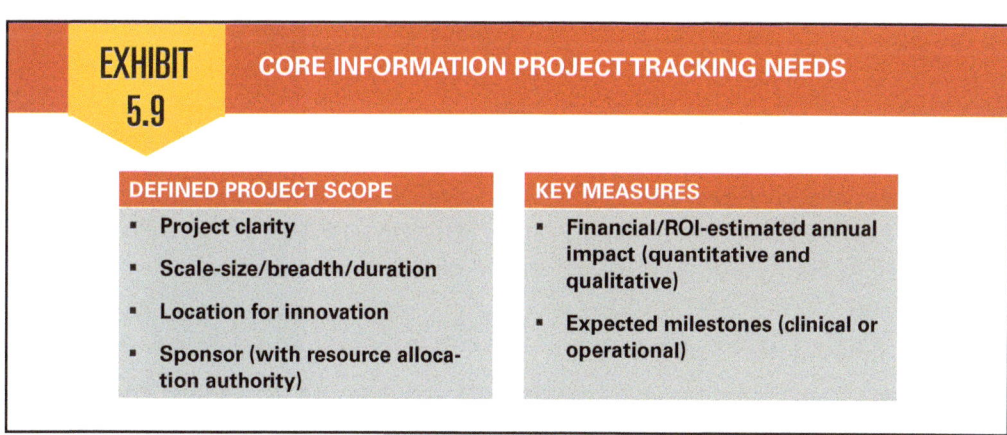

EXHIBIT 5.9 — CORE INFORMATION PROJECT TRACKING NEEDS

DEFINED PROJECT SCOPE	KEY MEASURES
▪ Project clarity	▪ Financial/ROI-estimated annual impact (quantitative and qualitative)
▪ Scale-size/breadth/duration	
▪ Location for innovation	▪ Expected milestones (clinical or operational)
▪ Sponsor (with resource allocation authority)	

* These standards are based on the 2019 *Magnet® Application Manual*. For Magnet Recognition Program® updates and developments, please refer to https://www.nursingworld.org/organizational-programs/magnet/magnet-manual-updates/

Key measures related to financial returns and project milestones are documented in business case documents. The business case answers the question, "Why do this?" Each organization will have its own version of what is expected in a business case and approval processes required for levels of spending. A worthy business case template is a template that everyone will use, inputting data based on well-established template definitions that are consistently applied throughout the organization.

Typical sections in a business case template include project description, team members, expected timeline, summary statistics related to competition, risk, and investment decisions required to proceed. The business case helps focus the idea creator on what is relevant for the organization to consider about the proposed idea. Once the business case is approved based on key decision criteria that are understood and accepted by the team members and the organization, the idea then can move into pilot/prototyping for further evaluation. To track progress against projected returns and project achievements, the innovation idea is then placed into a project tracking system. The system measures investments (budgeted to actual) and the project progress.

All resources associated with the project are tracked, and updates, revision notices, project activity updates, and milestone charts should be sent to each person involved on a project. However, refer to Table 5.1, indicator 3, Just-Enough-Structure, to be mindful of balancing too much with too little information. Just as too little information makes team members feel left out, an abundance of information can serve to undermine your team's engagement with a project.

There is not a "best" way to establish your tracking system; there are numerous toolkits, exemplars, and resources that you can access to determine what will work best for you and your organization. If you work within a large or multisite hospital system, it is likely that you will already have tools available to help you set up your innovation model and tracking system.

Now imagine that you have selected and implemented your innovation model, that you are well prepared with a detailed innovation strategy plan, and that your tracking and data collection system is in place. What should you do next?

You need to prepare yourself for setbacks, challenges, and failure.

NAVIGATING SETBACKS AND FAILURES

On average, 40% of innovations fail,[42] so give yourself time to fail fast and to regroup to redesign your innovation, or to pursue other innovation ideas. Dr. Dave Richards, innovation expert, evaluated reasons for innovation failures; his work identifies 36 organizational, internal, and external factors affecting innovation success.[43] *Organizational barriers* include characteristics such as lacking an innovation agenda, strategies without an articulated purpose, working in silos, culture of blame and fear of failure, and lacking competence to carry out innovation. *Internal process barriers* encompass items such as unclear goals, projects under-resourced to achieve a goal, ineffective or no executive sponsor, misguided teamwork practices, lacking design thinking processes, and failure to quit when a project will not work. *External barriers* are influences such as disengaged sales channels and marketing teams, underestimating competitors, lack of adequate market research to target customers, and using misguided business models that are not supported by regulatory or industry conditions.

Other innovation industry research on implementation barriers from the Boston Consulting Group and McKinsey & Company supports Dr. Richards's conclusions. (See https://www.bcg.com/perspectives.aspx and https://www.mckinsey.com/insights/mckinsey_quarterly for a variety of innovation study reports).

EXERCISE 5.3	ASSESSING THE ORGANIZATIONAL ENVIRONMENT

- What cultural values do you think are needed to support innovation in your organization?
- Refer to the values you identified in Exercise 3.1 (see pg. 76). Do the values support innovation?
- As you identify your approach to innovation, consider what top five key failure points listed in Exhibit 5.10 will most significantly impact your efforts. How will you mitigate these risks?

EXHIBIT 5.10

EXAMPLES OF KEY INNOVATION POINTS

ORGANIZATIONAL	PROCESS	EXTERNAL
Channel effectiveness is diminished	Customer-focused feedback is not considered	Strategy to leverage brand equity is missing
Competencies are lacking	Evidence-based processes to evaluate progress are missing	Competitive advantages are not defined
Culture risk, reward, teams, collaboration are misaligned	Feedback used to refine/re-engineer projects is lacking/inconsistent	Customer targets are unclear
Customer focus is missing	Measurement systems and progress timelines are inadequate or missing	Industry trajectory is not available/unclear
Decision-making/action orientation is diminished	Partnership processes are not in place	Industry shifts (channel, customers, competitors) are unclear
Failure orientation is avoided	Processes to streamline time to market, decision-making, planning, and execution are lacking	Market scans are not available/minimal
Intellectual property policies and processes are missing	Processes to evaluate technology opportunities are misaligned/not available	Market disruptions are not considered and/or acted upon
Return-on-investment strategies are unclear	Processes to launch prototypes or projects are missing	Partners—failure to mobilize external opportunities

Now that you know what is included in an innovation model, let's look at a few models that today are propelling healthcare innovations and investments.

WHAT DOES AN INNOVATION MODEL LOOK LIKE?

The ANA Enterprise Innovation Framework allows nurses and colleagues to explore, create, and implement ideas that lead to better patient care. ANA leverages the power of many through partner collaborations by engaging innovators in a variety of ways—innovation is not a "one size fits all" process. ANA's innovation tactics reach potential innovators using a diverse range of initiatives such as those presented in Exhibit 5.11.

Each ANA innovation model leverages different processes depending on the outcomes to be achieved. Structures to lead initiatives also vary depending on collaborative partners, group size, and awards. For instance, the HIMSS-ANA Nurse Pitch™ was launched at the HIMSS 2019 conference, with cash prize awards for first-, second-, and third-place winners. It was designed as a 150-person luncheon with a two-hour pitch presentation. There

EXHIBIT
5.11

ANA ENTERPRISE INNOVATION MODELS

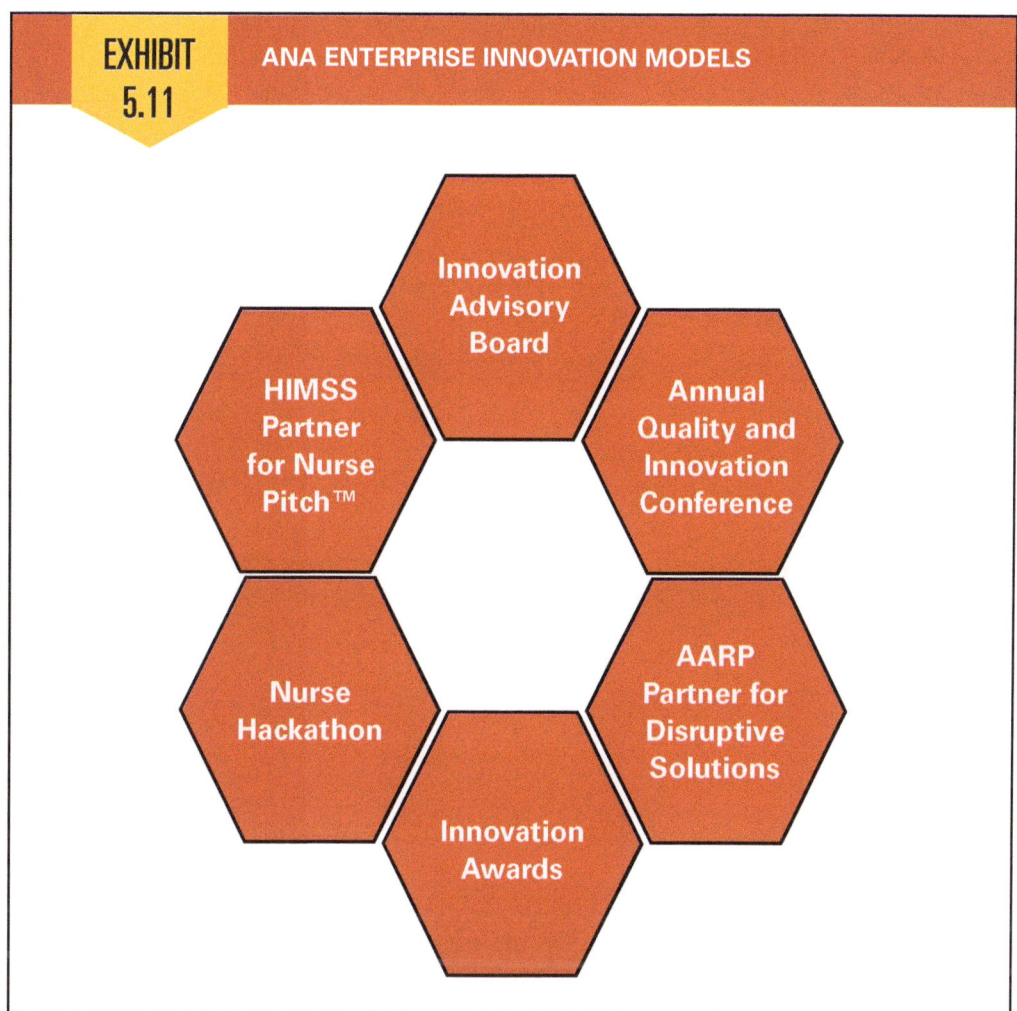

were two phases in the selection of candidates to present on the HIMSS19 Pitch Stage. First, applications were submitted from organizations seeking "pre-seed" and "series A" funding. Specific criteria and proposed items for inclusion with the initial submission were published with the application process. A formal application was submitted to the organizer, who recruited virtual panel judges. A virtual review process resulted in the selection of round-two candidates, who were invited to compete for the innovation prize awards at HIMSS2019.

ANA team members collaborated with partners to create a reference tool, *The Innovation Road Map: A Guide for Nurse Leaders*. The road map is supplemented with a detailed guide that provides recommendations for implementing innovation processes within an organization. The map and guide can be accessed at https://www.nursingworld.org/globalassets/ana /innovation-road-map-infographic.pdf.

The ANCC has established an innovation definition that is used to guide Magnet Recognition Program® standards and evaluation criteria for model component New Knowledge, Innovations & Improvements. The ANCC's Magnet® Model definition is as follows:[39]

> **Innovation is the application of creativity or problem solving that results in a widely adopted strategy, product, or service that meets a need in a new and different way. Innovations are about improvement in quality, cost effectiveness, or efficiency.**

Source: 2019 Magnet Application Manual, p. 161

The Magnet Model definition aligns with measures used to collect GII country index scores. Both models focus on meeting a need in a new and different way that results in a return on investment for resources committed. The implementation of new knowledge and innovations as defined by the Magnet Recognition Program® targets efforts in six core nursing activities (Exhibit 5.12).

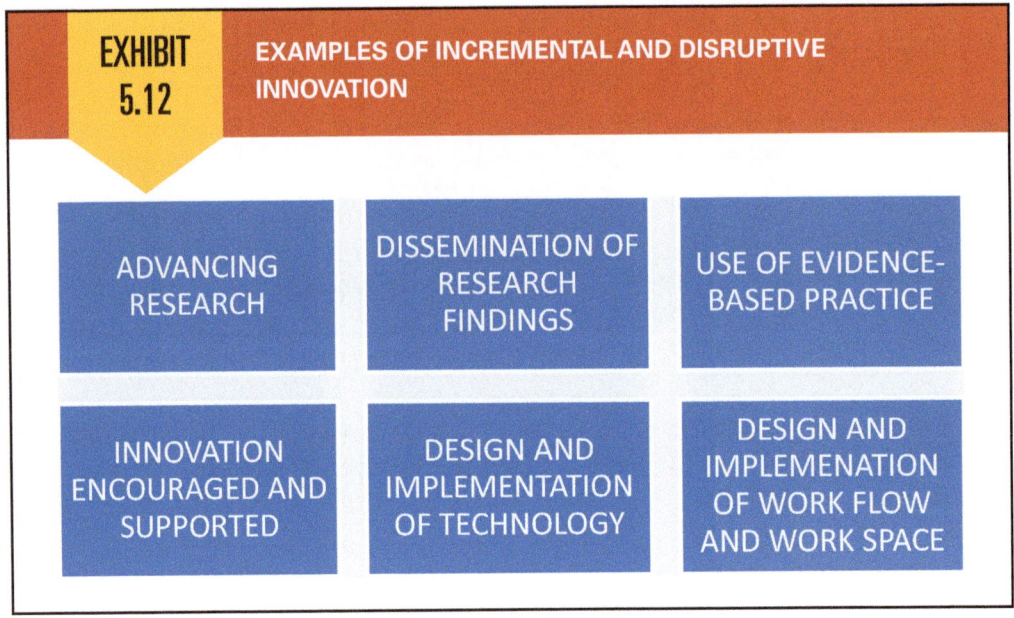

EXHIBIT 5.12 — EXAMPLES OF INCREMENTAL AND DISRUPTIVE INNOVATION

ADVANCING RESEARCH	DISSEMINATION OF RESEARCH FINDINGS	USE OF EVIDENCE-BASED PRACTICE
INNOVATION ENCOURAGED AND SUPPORTED	DESIGN AND IMPLEMENTATION OF TECHNOLOGY	DESIGN AND IMPLEMENATION OF WORK FLOW AND WORK SPACE

In 2003, Kaiser Permanente established the Innovation Consultancy group to bring new ideas, methods, and ways of working to the organization and to improve patient care. The team organizes its consultation services around this model.[44] The group describes itself as "a first-of-its-kind experiment to explore the value of human-centered design in health care."

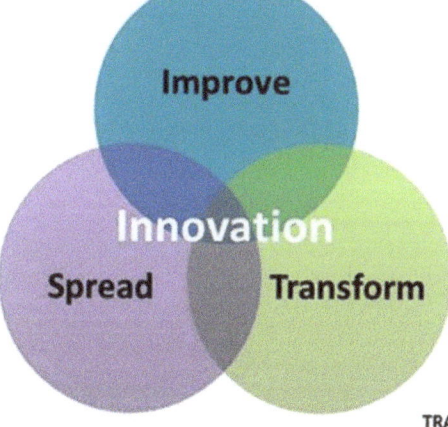

IMPROVE
Activities that solve problems or improve a current process, technology, or architectural design

SPREAD
Trainings, simulations or re-enactments that enable the spread or diffusion of practices or ideas

TRANSFORM
Sometimes called disruptive, these innovations help deliver health and wellness in new ways

Source: Used with permission of Kaiser Permanente, Garfield Innovation Center.

A critical step in an innovation initiative is to identify the cultural, process, and external issues that can sabotage your efforts.

Innovation barriers and key failure traits can be managed to reduce impacts on innovation efforts. Team members and innovation project sponsors need to plan in advance how they will navigate cultural and process challenges.

> **It is not enough to bring in experts, strike at the ripe time, encourage creativity and freewheeling experiments, hold a tolerance for mistakes and failures, play, and cultivate intuition and curiosity. To succeed you must master the activities required to create the kind of products and services that get traction and grow.**
>
> *—Seth Kahan, Innovation Expert*[45]

The opening pages of Step 5 provided you an overview of innovation fundamentals and presented examples of tools that can help you manage innovation projects. Start your innovation journey with a clearly defined innovation process that includes:

- Articulation of the problem or opportunity being pursued,

- Transparent decision criteria for project selections,

- Data monitoring capabilities, and

- Return on investment targets and project milestones.

Your innovation process must be supported by effective innovation leadership and a culture that seeks out innovation as an expected way to conduct business. Even with this in place, given that many projects fail, you need to prepare yourself to identify and manage innovation barriers.

In Step 6 we will look at how Artificial Intelligence and big data are affecting healthcare innovation.

REFERENCES

1. Śledzik, K. (2013). Schumpeter's view on innovation and entrepreneurship. *Management Trends in Theory and Practice.* DOI: 10.2139/ssrn.2257783.

2. Cornell University, INSEAD, and WIPO. (2019). *The Global Innovation Index 2019: Creating healthy lives—The future of medical innovation.* Ithaca, Fontainebleau, and Geneva: Author.

3. OECD. (2018). *Oslo manual 2018: Guidelines for collecting, reporting and using data on innovation.* Retrieved from http://www.oecd.org/sti/oslo-manual-2018-9789264304604-en.htm

4. McCarthy, N. (2019, July 25). The world's most innovative countries. Statistica. Retrieved from https://www.statista.com/chart/18804/rankings-of-the-global-innovation-index/

5. Khedkar, P., & Sahay, D. (2019). Chapter 3: Trends in healthcare and medical innovation. In: *The Global Innovation Index 2019: Creating healthy lives—The future of medical innovation.* Ithaca, Fontainebleau, and Geneva: Cornell University, INSEAD, and WIPO.

6. Christensen, C. M., Bohmer, R., & Kenagy, J. (2000, September). Will disruptive innovations cure health care? *Harvard Business Review,* 1–10.

7. Goozner, M. (2015, January 24). Boosting the right kind of innovation. *Modern Healthcare.* Retrieved from http://www.modernhealthcare.com/article/20150124/MAGAZINE/301249984

8. Dreamit. (2018, April 13). On the rise: Digital health startups see uptick in year-over-year venture funding for Q1 2018. Retrieved from https://www.dreamit.com/journal/2018/4/13/on-the-rise-digital-health -startups-see-uptick-in-year-over-year-venture-funding-for-q1-2018

9. Tindera, M. (2018, December 27). These 10 VC firms made the most investments in healthcare startups this year. *Forbes*. Retrieved from https://www.forbes.com/sites/michelatindera/2018/12/27/these-10-vc -firms-made-the-most-investments-in-healthcare-startups-this-year

10. Tahir, D. (2015). Innovations: Testing a digital pillbox to improve medication compliance. *Modern Healthcare*. Retrieved from http://www.modernhealthcare.com/article/20150516/MAGAZINE /305169971?

11. Associated Press. (2015). Software turns smartphones into tools for medical research. *Modern Healthcare*. Retrieved from http://www.modernhealthcare.com/article/20150727/NEWS/307279980?

12. Evans, M. (2015). Innovations: Using software tools to strengthen bonds between nurses and patients. *Modern Healthcare*. Retrieved from http://www.modernhealthcare.com/article/20150530 /MAGAZINE/305309975?

13. Deloitte Center for Health Solutions. (2015). *The convergence of health care trends: Innovation strategies for emerging opportunities*. Retrieved from http://www2.deloitte.com/us/en/pages/life-sciences -and-health-care/articles/convergence-health-care-trends.html

14. Centers for Medicare & Medicaid Services. (2014, December). *CMS Innovation Center: Report to Congress*. Retrieved from http://innovation.cms.gov/Files/reports/RTC-12-2014.pdf

15. Centers for Medicare & Medicaid Services. (2015). National health expenditure data. Retrieved from https://www.cms.gov/Research-Statistics-Data-and-Systems/Statistics-Trends-and-Reports/National HealthExpendData/NationalHealthAccountsProjected.html

16. Agency for Healthcare Research and Quality. (2010). *2010 National healthcare quality report*. Rockville, MD: Author.

17. Kamal, R., Sawyer, B., & McDermott, D. (2019, March 12). An annual percentage point difference in growth rates makes a very large difference in spending over time. Peterson-Kaiser Health System Tracker. Retrieved from https://www.healthsystemtracker.org/chart-collection/much-health-spending -expected-grow

18. BCG Henderson Institute. (2017). *Health care's value problem—And how to fix it: Simple rules for delivering improved health outcomes at lower cost*. Retrieved from http://image-src.bcg.com/Images/BCG _VBHC_WebV12_tcm30-174204.pdf

19. Wicklund, E. (2013, July 31). Glassomic looks to unlock the potential of Google Glass. *mHealthNews*. Retrieved from http://www.mhealthnews.com/blog/digital-health-moving-toward-healthcare-revolution

20. Heinzman, A. (2019, February 14). Google Glass isn't dead; it's the future of industry. Blog post. Retrieved from https://www.howtogeek.com/400963/google-glass-isnt-dead-and-its-the-future -of-industry/

21. CBINSIGHTS. (n.d.). How Google plans to use AI to reinvent the $3 trillion US healthcare industry. Retrieved from https://www.cbinsights.com/research/report/google-strategy-healthcare/

22. Su, J. (2018, September 14). Apple Watch 4 is now an FDA class 2 medical device: Detects fall, irregular heart rhythm. *Forbes*. Retrieved from https://www.forbes.com/sites/jeanbaptiste/2018/09/14/apple -watch-4-is-now-an-fda-class-2-medical-device-detects-falls-irregular-heart-rhythm/#2f781f207135

23. Haven. (n.d.). Vision. Retrieved from https://havenhealthcare.com/vision

24. Safavi, K., & Dare, F. (2018, April 3). Virtual health care could save the U.S. Billions each year. *Harvard Business Review*.

25. ATA. (2019). *2019 State of the states report: Coverage and reimbursement*. Retrieved from https://www .americantelemed.org/initiatives/2019-state-of-the-states-report-coverage-and-reimbursement/

26. Farr, C. (2019, May 13). The inside story of why Amazon bought PillPack in its effort to crack the $500 bil- lion prescription market. CNBC. Retrieved from https://www.cnbc.com/2019/05/10/why-amazon-bought -pillpack-for-753-million-and-what-happens-next.html

27. Madara, J. L. (2019, March 4). Shooting for the moon: Rules for audacious innovation in healthcare. Health2047. Retrieved from https://health2047.com/2019/03/04/shooting-for-the-moon-rules-for-audacious -innovation-in-healthcare/

28. Beckland, R. (2015, August 6). Digital health: Moving towards a healthcare revolution. *mHealthNews*. Retrieved from http://www.mhealthnews.com/blog/digital-health-moving-toward-healthcare-revolution

29. Wicklund, E. (2015, January 16). Google Glass reaches a crossroads. *mHealthNews*. Retrieved from http://www.healthcareitnews.com/blog/google-glass-reaches-crossroads

30. Google Glass Apps. (n.d.). Google Glass application list. Retrieved from http://glass-apps.org/google -glass-application-list

31. Robert Wood Johnson Foundation. (2015). *Discovering new ideas*. Retrieved from http://www.rwjf.org /en/how-we-work/discovering-new-ideas.html

32. Everett, L. Q., & Sitterding, M. C. (2013). Building a culture of innovation by maximizing the role of the RN. *Nursing Administration Quarterly*, *37*(3), 194–202.

33. Cass, D. (2013, September 25). How to get health care innovations to take off. *Harvard Business Review*. Retrieved from https://hbr.org/2013/09/how-to-get-health-care-innovations-to-take-off

34. Pisano, G. P. (2015, June). You need an innovation strategy. *Harvard Business Review*. Retrieved from https://hbr.org/2015/06/you-need-an-innovation-strategy

35. Malloch, K., & Mazurek Melnyk, B. (2013). Developing high-level change and innovation agents. *Nursing Administration Quarterly*, *37*(1), 60–66.

36. Hunter, S. T., Ligon, G. S., & Myer, A. T. (2011). Paradoxes of leading innovative endeavors: Summary, solutions, and future directions. *Psychology of Aesthetics, Creativity, and the Arts*, *5*(1), 54–66.

37. Dyer, J. H., Gregersen, H. B., & Christensen, C. M. (2009). The innovator's DNA (cover story). *Harvard Business Review*, *87*, 60–67.

38. Bellman, G. M. & Ryan, K. (2009). *Extraordinary groups: How ordinary teams achieve amazing results*. San Francisco: Jossey-Bass.

39. American Nurses Credentialing Center. (2019). *Magnet Recognition Program®: Application manual.* Silver Spring, MD: Author.

40. Glassman, K., & Rosenfeld, P. (2015*). Data makes the difference: The smart nurse's handbook for using data to improve care.* Silver Spring, MD: Nursesbooks.org.

41. Institute for Healthcare Improvement (IHI). (2015). *Innovation quality project summary sheet multi-project tracking tool.* Retrieved from http://www.ihi.org/resources/Pages/Tools/InnovationQuality ProjectSummarySheetMultiProjectTrackingTool.aspx

42. Castellion, G., & Markham, S. K. (2013). Perspective: New product failure rates: Influence of *argumentum ad populum* and self-interest. *Journal of Product Innovation Management, 30*(5), 976–979.

43. Balmaekers, H. (2014). *The one word answer to why innovation fails.* Retrieved from http://www .innovationmanagement.se/2014/09/22/the-one-word-answer-to-why-innovation-fails/

44. Tonges, M., & Ray, J. D. (2015) Creating a culture of rapid change adoption: Implementing an innovations unit. *Journal of Nursing Administration, 45*(7/8), 384–390.

45. Kahan, S. (2013). *Visionary leadership.* Retrieved from http://www.visionaryleadership.com/site/getting -innovation-right.php

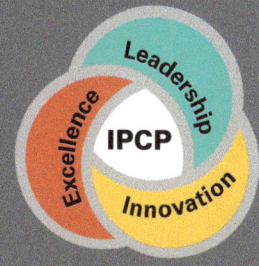

AI AND BIG DATA—
OPPORTUNITY OR DANGER?

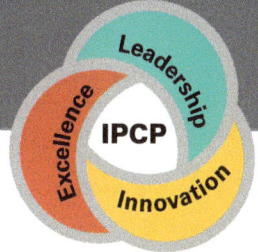

AI AND BIG DATA— OPPORTUNITY OR DANGER?

All the tools, techniques, and technology in the world are nothing without the head, heart, and hands to use them wisely, kindly and mindfully.

—Rasheed Ogunlaru, Life Coach

AI AND BIG DATA—WHAT IS IT AND HOW IS IT CHANGING HEALTH CARE?

Today there is no doubt that health care is experiencing rapid transformations that are accelerated by technology advancements. Of significant impact are artificial intelligence (AI) and big data—technologies that have been in development for decades. Why are these technologies now front and center? Because significant improvements in internet deployment, hardware, software, and data science have provided opportunities to innovate new products and services. This step explores what AI and big data are and how these technologies are impacting decision-making.

RECOMMENDED READING

Robert, N. (2019). How artificial intelligence is changing nursing. *Journal of Nursing Management*. https://journals.lww.com/nursingmanagement/Fulltext/2019/09000/How_artificial_intelligence_is_changing_nursing.8.aspx

Deloitte Life Sciences and Health Care. (2019). 2019 Global health care outlook: Shaping the future. Retrieved from https://www2.deloitte.com/content/dam/Deloitte/global/Documents/Life-Sciences-Health-Care/gx-lshc-hc-outlook-2019.pdf

Draper, R. (2018, February). They are watching you. National Geographic, 30–65.

THE CONNECTED WORLD

Step 5: Innovation highlighted that 2019 global investments in health care are estimated to reach $177 billion, with the technology sector driving a significant portion of global investment activity. In the United States, 2019 healthcare investments are estimated to exceed $28 billion. What is driving investment in healthcare technology?

Digital Reach

People today have more access to information, data, and applications that impact personal and professional life—technology innovations dominate how we live, who we communicate with, and how we are connected to multitudes of daily life endeavors. According to Statistica, today the World Wide Web provides access to over 4.3 billion global consumers, which represents 56% of the world's population.[1] Pew's Spring 2018 Global Attitudes Survey estimates that there are about 5 million mobile devices in use, with 50% of the devices being smartphones.[2] In the United States, 2019 Pew Research Center surveys indicate that 90% of U.S. adults aged 18 and over have access to the internet, with the studies suggesting that multiple factors such as age, education level, and income impact internet usage (see Exhibit 6.1).[3]

The Pew research found significant differences in internet use by age, with 73% of those aged 65 and over—a cohort with the lowest use across all adults aged 18 and over—used the internet in 2019. Comparatively, those aged 18–29 reported 100% use of the internet. Those with less than a high school education reported 71% internet usage, while 98%

of college graduates claimed internet usage. Whereas 82% of individuals with less than $30,000 annual income reported internet usage, 98% of those earning $75,000 or more used the internet. Of those adults reporting internet use, about 75% have digital broadband access from home.[3]

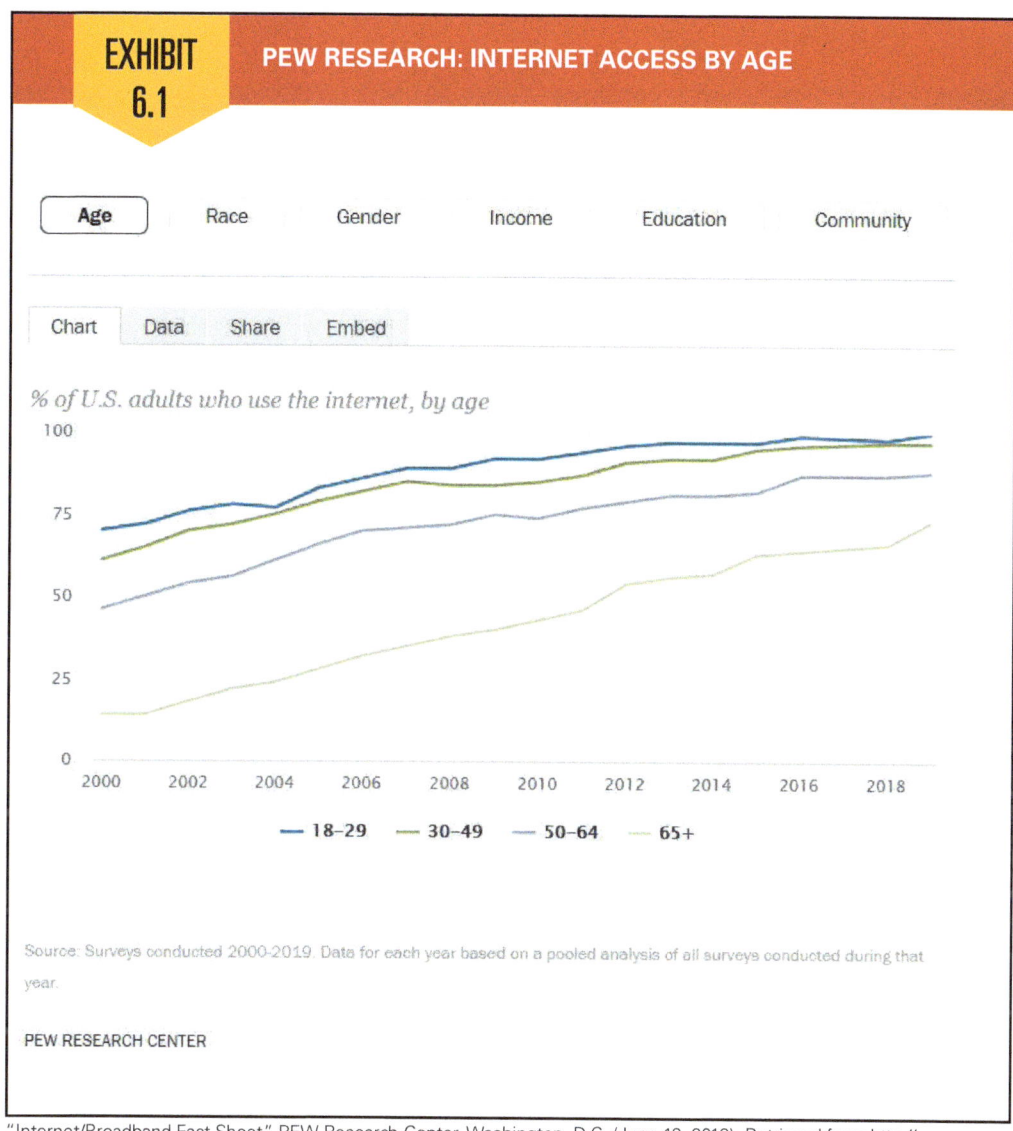

EXHIBIT 6.1 — PEW RESEARCH: INTERNET ACCESS BY AGE

Age   Race   Gender   Income   Education   Community

Chart   Data   Share   Embed

% of U.S. adults who use the internet, by age

— 18–29   — 30–49   — 50–64   — 65+

Source: Surveys conducted 2000-2019. Data for each year based on a pooled analysis of all surveys conducted during that year.

PEW RESEARCH CENTER

"Internet/Broadband Fact Sheet." PEW Research Center, Washington, D.C. (June 12, 2019). Retrieved from http://www. pewinternet.org/fact-sheet/internet-broadband

People continue to use multiple devices to access applications and information, which requires companies to invest in numerous technologies that work across a variety of platforms. In the United States, 95% of adults report having a cell phone, with 77% of cell phones identified as smartphones.[4] Smartphone use is not equal across generations—92% of millennials (those born 1981–96) own a smartphone while only 30% of the silent generation (born 1945 and earlier) report smartphone ownership.[5]

For those aged 18 and over, Exhibit 6.2 displays Pew research regarding technologies used to access a variety of digital applications.[4] As with smartphone usage, age does influence technology use. Pew findings reveal age differences in tablet ownership with 54% of millennials owning a device, which is nearly equal to the 52% baby boomer ownership rate but significantly differs from the silent generation. Only 25% of silent generation adults aged 74 and older report owning a tablet.[5]

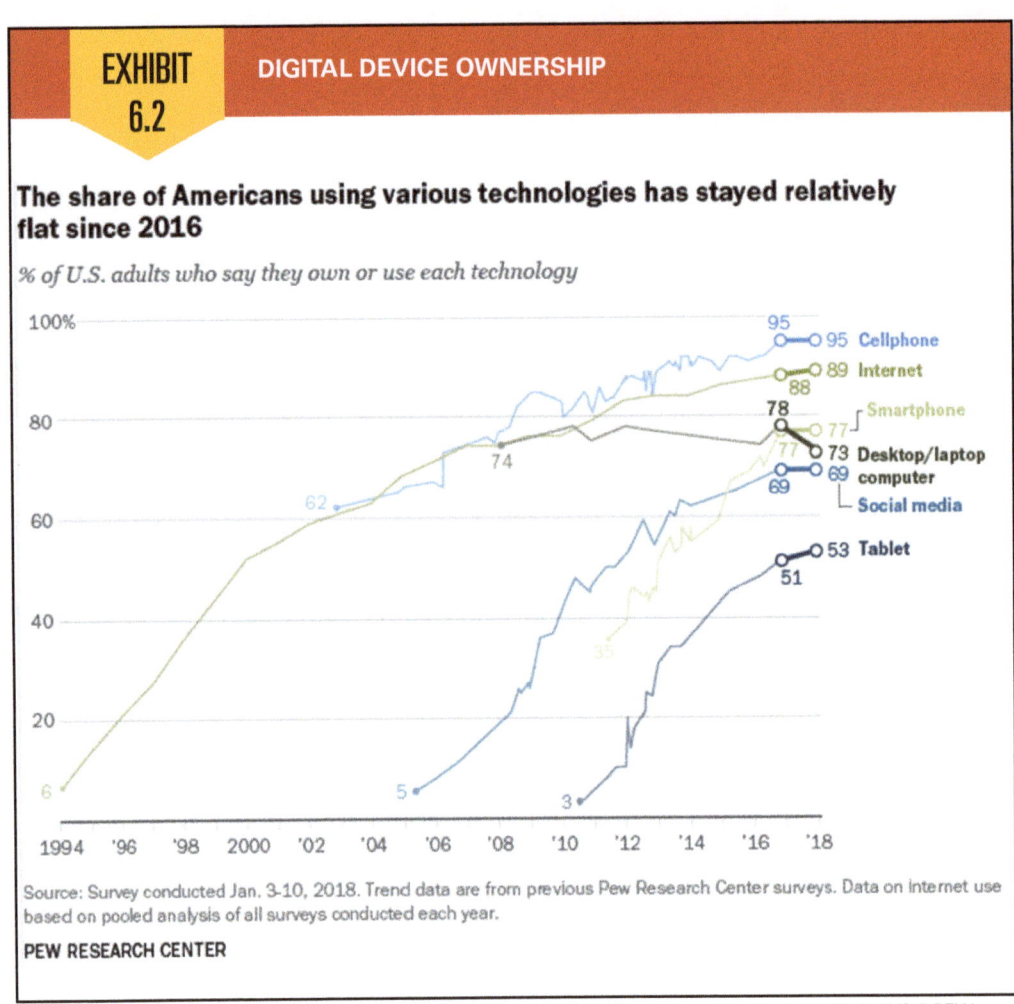

EXHIBIT 6.2 DIGITAL DEVICE OWNERSHIP

The share of Americans using various technologies has stayed relatively flat since 2016

% of U.S. adults who say they own or use each technology

Source: Survey conducted Jan. 3-10, 2018. Trend data are from previous Pew Research Center surveys. Data on internet use based on pooled analysis of all surveys conducted each year.

PEW RESEARCH CENTER

Jingjing, Jiang. "Millennials Stand Out for their Technology Use, But Older Generations Also Embrace Digital Life." PEW Research Center, Washington, D.C. (May 2, 2018). Retrieved from https://www.pewresearch.org/fact-tank/2019/09/09/us-generations-technology-use/

The bottom line is that the majority of people in the United States are digitally connected in some way, and this is contributing to the growth in applications, artificial intelligence, and big data innovations. As more people connect through technology, they create data that are then collected by various technology companies that then use the information as inputs into the development of new products and services. This drives an endless circle of digital innovation. While there is much controversy regarding the collection of personal information that sometimes impinges on privacy boundaries, it is not expected that data collection and aggregation efforts by technology providers will stop.

Applications

Healthcare applications are a leading vertical in the digital revolution, with healthcare data accounting for about a third of the world's data.[6] In Step 5: Innovation, healthcare applications from Amazon, Apple, Google, and Microsoft were highlighted. According to data collected in Meeker's *Internet Trends 2018 Report*,[7] Deloitte found that six of the top ten technology companies had entered health care. New entrants are transforming health care, and new partnerships such as Health2047 are redefining roles of existing players in the healthcare market.

Data are not only generated in hospital delivery systems. Today, consumers and manufacturers are using sensors to transmit data to other machines or to people. It is estimated that globally 23+ million Internet of Things (IoT) devices connect through the World Wide Web with applications such as smart watches, smart cars, medical monitoring apps and devices, Alexa, Nest, and Ring. The number of connected devices is expected to grow to over 75 billion by 2025.[8,9] Given the endless cycle of worldwide digital data creation, the IoT market is predicted to have continued spending. According to the Grand View Research Report, the global IoT Healthcare Market will grow to $534.3 billion by 2025. Key drivers of the projected growth are the use of IoT to manage chronic diseases using remote monitoring and new platforms that offer real-time data and analytics support.[10]

Is the healthcare industry ready to embrace connected devices? Based on predictions by the IBM Institute for Business Value and Deloitte Consulting, over the next decade deployment of medical IoT should reach "50 billion devices connected to clinicians, health systems, patients, and to each other."[11]

Findings from the Deloitte Center for Health Solutions 2018 Surveys of Physicians and Health Care Consumers indicates that 57% of consumers would be willing to try virtual office visits (which are counted in Deloitte IoT figures), while 23% of consumers had already experienced a virtual visit with a physician or nurse. However, there seems to be a gap in consumer willingness versus clinician readiness to respond to this technology advancement—over 50% of consumers with health tracking devices reported sharing the information with their physician, while only 9% of doctors had implemented systems to integrate data gathered from patient remote devices.[12]

IoMT is considered a subset of IoT devices that employ medical sensors in a variety of devices to collect, analyze, and send patient and medical information through the web. Devices that allow for remote patient monitoring of heart and diabetic patients, collection of hospital bed stats, pill dispensing and pill reminder monitoring, and applications such as telemedicine support the delivery of health care today. The Gartner Group's *Top 10 Strategic Technology Trends for 2019 Report* identifies artificial intelligence (AI) technologies today that automate or augment IoT/IoMT devices and predicts the trend will continue as AI capabilities improve.

How are technology companies organizing products and services to support health care? Exhibit 6.3 highlights how new entrants are connecting to the healthcare market.

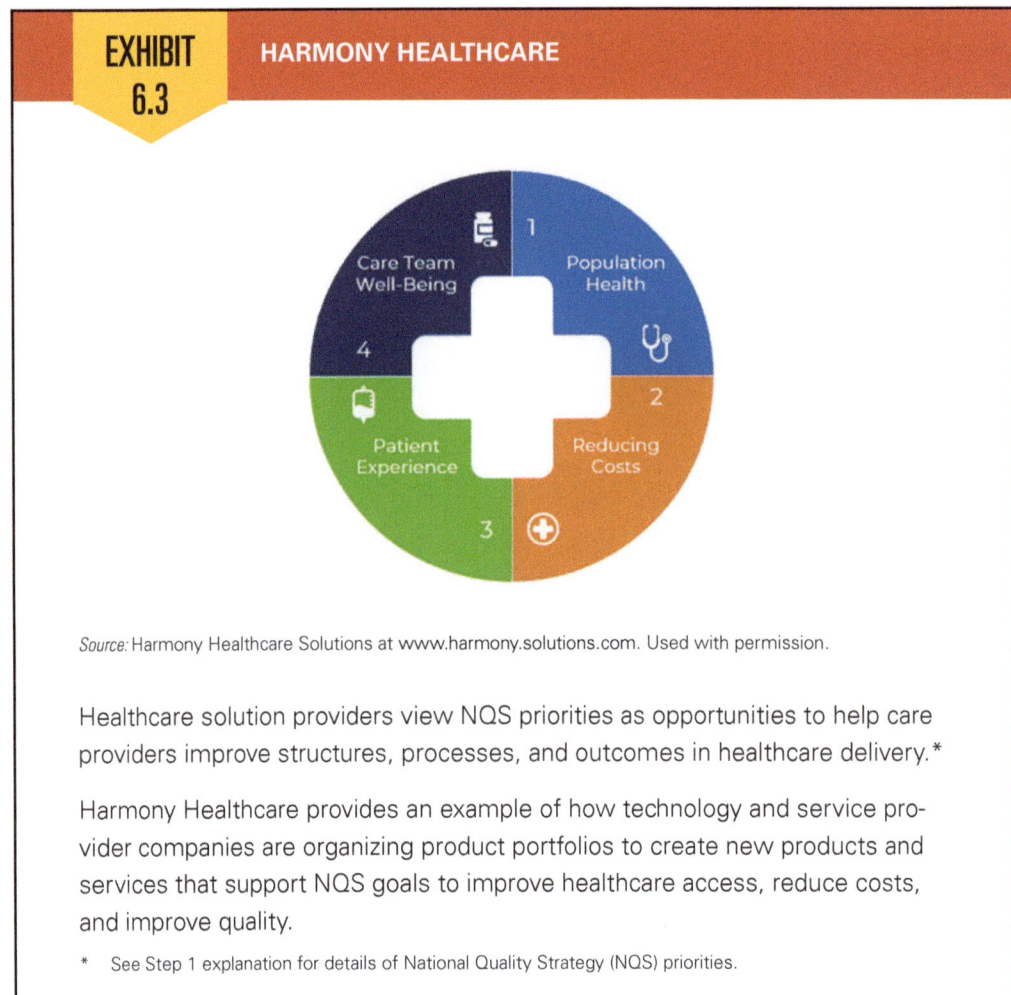

EXHIBIT 6.3

HARMONY HEALTHCARE

Source: Harmony Healthcare Solutions at www.harmony.solutions.com. Used with permission.

Healthcare solution providers view NQS priorities as opportunities to help care providers improve structures, processes, and outcomes in healthcare delivery.*

Harmony Healthcare provides an example of how technology and service provider companies are organizing product portfolios to create new products and services that support NQS goals to improve healthcare access, reduce costs, and improve quality.

* See Step 1 explanation for details of National Quality Strategy (NQS) priorities.

A 2013 report by EMC and IDC research estimated that by 2020 the volume of healthcare data would swell to 2,314 exabytes. To help visualize what this means, IDC estimated that in 2020 to store this amount of data using 2013 storage capabilities available on tablet computers, you would need to stack the tablets 82,000 miles high, which is about a third of the way to the moon.[13] If we reached 2020 figures, globally we would not have enough capacity to store all healthcare data. VisualCapital estimated that we would need to increase storage capacity by 2.5 times.[14] This data projection was published in 2013. Technology providers took advantage of identified market needs and this, along with advances in technologies, contributed to the healthcare sector technology explosion.

With this amount of data, the challenge becomes, what do we do with the data we have collected and how do we use it to improve the delivery of health care? This is where AI and big data technologies are helping drive transformations and solutions in health care.

BIG DATA: EXACTLY WHAT IS IT?

It seems that the term *big data* has differing expert perspectives on what it actually means. Jenna Dutcher of Berkeley surveyed 40 data experts to see if a common definition could be derived.[15] Unfortunately the experts could not agree, so here are a few definitions that reflect the state of big data (see Exhibit 6.4).

Why such confusion over big data? Because technology advances continue to accelerate at amazing rates, spawning a race to create new platforms, tools, and processes. It is difficult to pinpoint what "big" means—is it today's definition or tomorrow's prediction? So, when you are asked about your organization's big data innovation projects, start your conversation with a clarification about what is being referred to.

EXHIBIT 6.4

WHAT IS BIG DATA?

'Big Data' is that everything we do is increasingly leaving a digital trace (or data), which we (and others) can use and analyze. Big data therefore refers to that data being collected and our ability to make use of it.

—Bernard Marr, leading data expert[16]

[Big data is an] umbrella term that means a lot of different things, but to me, it means the possibility of doing extraordinary things using modern machine learning techniques on digital data. Whether it is predicting illness, the weather, the spread of infectious diseases, or what you will buy next, it offers a world of possibilities for improving people's lives.

—Shashi Upadhyay, founder of Lattice Engines[15]

Despite its complexity, the U.S. big-data industry continues to grow (as shown in Exhibit 6.5).[17] Companies are seeking a competitive advantage with data. In health care, data-driven organizations are using data to identify population health needs, improve effectiveness and efficiency of service delivery, predict disease epidemics, and improve quality of life indicators for patients.[18,19]

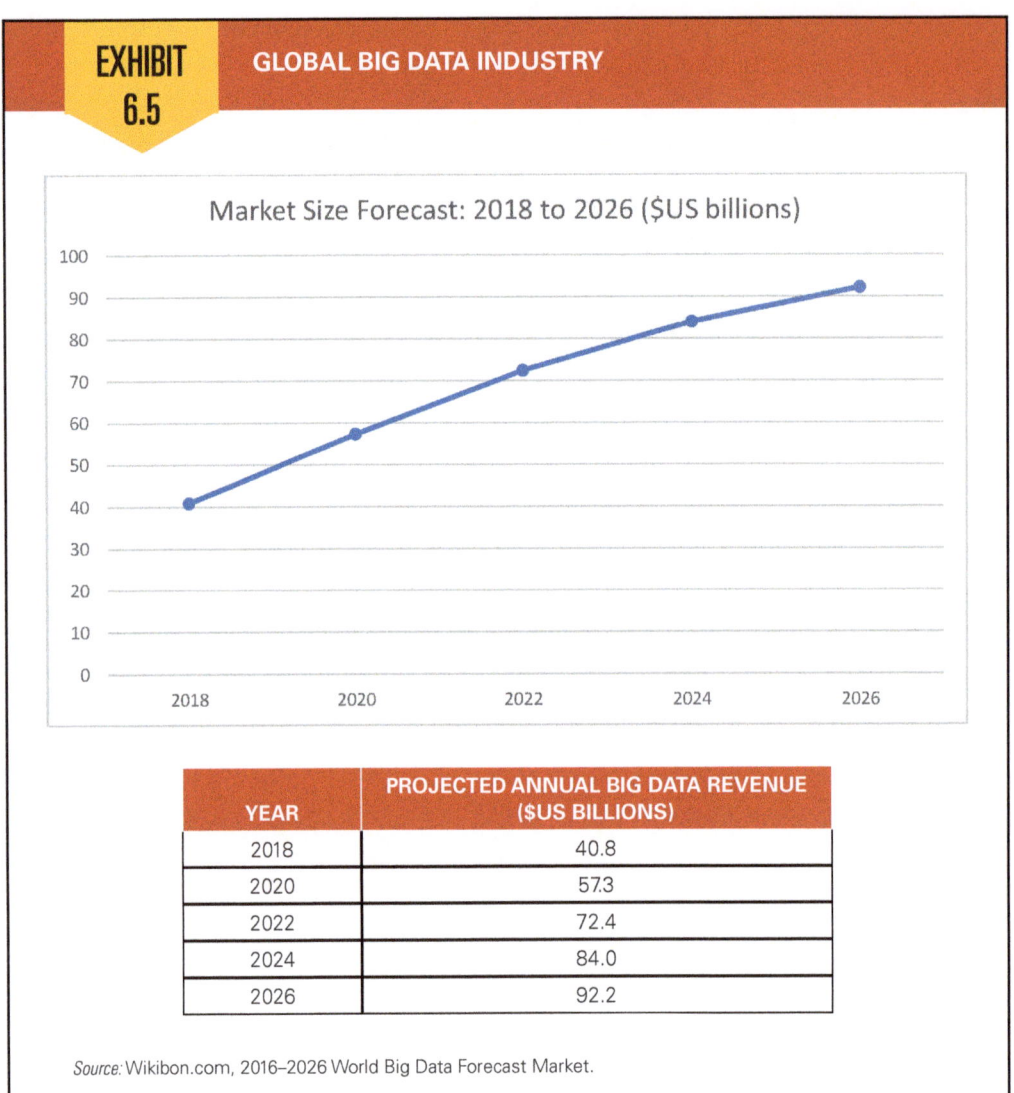

EXHIBIT 6.5	GLOBAL BIG DATA INDUSTRY

Market Size Forecast: 2018 to 2026 ($US billions)

YEAR	PROJECTED ANNUAL BIG DATA REVENUE ($US BILLIONS)
2018	40.8
2020	57.3
2022	72.4
2024	84.0
2026	92.2

Source: Wikibon.com, 2016–2026 World Big Data Forecast Market.

WHY IS BIG DATA IMPORTANT?

Today, innovation is tightly coupled with data and emerging technologies. Collaborations and alliances are being created to leverage scarce data-scientist resources and to gain experience in the application of big data to solve real-world problems. Alliances between companies such as Apple and IBM[20,21] have been created to provide cloud-based analytic services and, over time, have extended the partnership into machine learning integrations. Collaborations in citywide data initiatives like the Pittsburg Health Data Alliance have surfaced,[22] as well as a $100+ million investment in the future of big data analytics from companies such as Deloitte Touche Inc. to form ConvergeHEALTH,[23] a company that specifically addresses big data needs in healthcare markets. In 2014, the National Institutes of Health awarded $32 million in grants through their Knowledge Initiative to support development of novel big data analytics and tools.[24] NIH has formed an Office of Data Science and Technology that in 2019 is funding 143 data science grants.[25] As the volume of data increases exponentially, funds are being poured into big data with hopes of discovering new ways to manage information while creating novel connections potentially leading to improved healthcare outcomes and delivery of healthcare services.

In 2014, IDC, a technology forecasting company, predicted that by 2020 digital information will grow to 40 zettabytes (one zettabyte is approximately one billion terabytes).[26] By 2020 every person will generate 1.7 megabytes of data in one second.[27] What are we doing to generate so much data? Every minute we send 204 million emails and 278 thousand tweets, and upload 200 thousand photos to Facebook and 100 hours of video to YouTube. And each day we query Google 3.5 billion times.[28] The generation of data in health care is exploding. Roski, Bo-Linn, and Andrews report that by 2020 healthcare data will equal about 25,000 petabytes of data, which would fill about 500 billion file cabinets.[26] The world is digitally engaged, and big data's job is to collect all that is known and combine those data in novel ways to uncover new insights about real-world problems.

The pursuit of big data in nursing is not new, and companies such as Microsoft are providing resources to ensure that the 29-million-strong global nursing professionals contributes to the evolution of healthcare technologies.[29] Since 2013, nursing leaders and nursing informatics specialists have been pursuing action plans to capture nursing information and associated patient outcomes for big data research. Data tools such as the Rothman Index capture nursing team impacts on patient care, with research confirming that nursing care does make a difference in patient outcomes.[30,31,46] Core requirements of ANCC's Magnet Recognition Program's® Model components *Empirical Outcomes* and *New Knowledge, Innovations, and Improvements* are focused on nursing's contribution to the design, implementation, and evaluation of data, and the use of information technology in achieving patient care outcomes. Big data efforts can be viewed as the next generation of technology and knowledge expansion driving changes in healthcare delivery.[32]

Table 6.1 provides a preview of big data innovation projects that have emerged and identifies the complexities required to implement big data solutions focused on patient healthcare needs.

Health care is seen as a place where big data can be used to address the pressures of new regulatory requirements, to data-mine patient medical records to answer best practice questions, and to identify opportunities to reduce healthcare costs.[38]

TABLE 6.1
BIG DATA PROJECTS IN HEALTH CARE

Analysis of patient records to predict future risk of metabolic syndrome.[33]	ConvergeHEALTH is providing support to help Intermountain Healthcare sort through two trillion medical records to derive medical insights.[23]
Apple and IBM have teamed up to explore integrating Apple Watch data with Watson's artificial intelligence capabilities.[20]	Uses of patient-generated data to conduct comparative effectiveness research.[35]
Using big data to manage high-risk and high-cost patients.[28]	Veterans Health Administration's journey collecting and using big data.[36]
Beth Israel Deaconess Medical Center's data growth and the management of big data in its academic institution.[34]	An exploration of big data to advance prediction, performance, and comparative effectiveness research to address patient population health and medical practice.[37]

EXERCISE 6.1   **EXPERIENCE DATA ANALYTICS**

IBM provides a free version of Cognos Analytics 11.1 to those interested in experimenting with analytical dashboards focused on answering business questions. The tool provides you an opportunity to upload data and experience processing of your data to derive unique insights and empirical outputs. To use the site, perform the following steps:

1. Go to https://www.ibm.com/products/cognos-analytics and watch the video overview.

2. Create your IBM ID at https://www.ibm.com/account/reg/us-en /signup?formid=urx-34710.

3. Use your ID to access the analytics site and begin with the videos that explain how the analytic engine works. Step-by-step tutorials can guide you through the big data experience using your own data.

ARTIFICIAL INTELLIGENCE AND COGNITIVE COMPUTING

There are many definitions used to describe artificial intelligence (AI). For this discussion, the definition of AI created by Deloitte, a recognized global leader in data and analytic services, will serve as a point of reference—"the theory and development of computer systems able to perform tasks that normally require human intelligence."[39]

AI comprises a variety of technologies and methodologies that work together to try to match or exceed human intelligence. AI requires massive amounts of data to generate results and is supported by big data initiatives. While not all big data projects use AI, AI must have big data sets in order to process information and generate outputs. What's the difference between big data and AI? A big data project can leverage traditional business intelligence (BI) tools that use statistical and analytical processes to generate predictive insights, and to conduct data mining activities that can lead to new knowledge about the data. BI tools are not "teaching" the software, so the software does not learn from data sets—it predicts from data sets provided to it. AI systems use data to gain knowledge and do generate new insights from data—the machine has the capacity to learn and adjust its processing algorithms and outputs as new data are presented to it.

Exhibit 6.6 provides an overview of the most commonly deployed technologies used by AI teams today. Artificial intelligence is a term that is often used and frequently misunderstood. You should think about AI as being a portfolio of technologies that serve different functions. AI spans multiple technologies that contain unique capabilities deployed in a variety of product and service offerings, with the selection of technology based on the type of problem being addressed. Common features of AI systems are systems that represent human intelligence capabilities to reason, plan, solve problems, conduct abstract reasoning, comprehend situations to resolve conflicts, and to learn from experience—traits that, according to research by Gottfredson and colleagues, define human intelligence. (See https://www.ncbi.nlm.nih.gov/pmc/articles/PMC3181994/ for a detailed overview of human intelligence and the brain.[40])

Cognitive computing is a term that captures capabilities frequently associated with AI technologies. Entities such as IBM, Deloitte, and other large-scale AI deployment experts often use AI and Cognitive Computing interchangeably, to describe computer functionality that mimics human capabilities. Definitions among industry experts vary as to what constitutes cognitive computing versus AI, with some citing AI outputs being distinguished by their ability to deliver definitive answers generated by a machine, versus cognitive computing systems that deliver reasoning and insights that are used to supplement human decision-making. The *2017 Deloitte Cognitive Survey* refers to cognitive technologies as "technologies that can perform and/or augment tasks, help better inform decisions, and create interactions that have traditionally required human intelligence, such as planning, reasoning from partial or uncertain information, and learning."[41] Whether you are seeking a decision to solve a problem or trying to gain insights about a problem, there are common features that comprise cognitive capabilities in computing systems.

EXHIBIT 6.6	COGNITIVE TECHNOLOGIES[39]

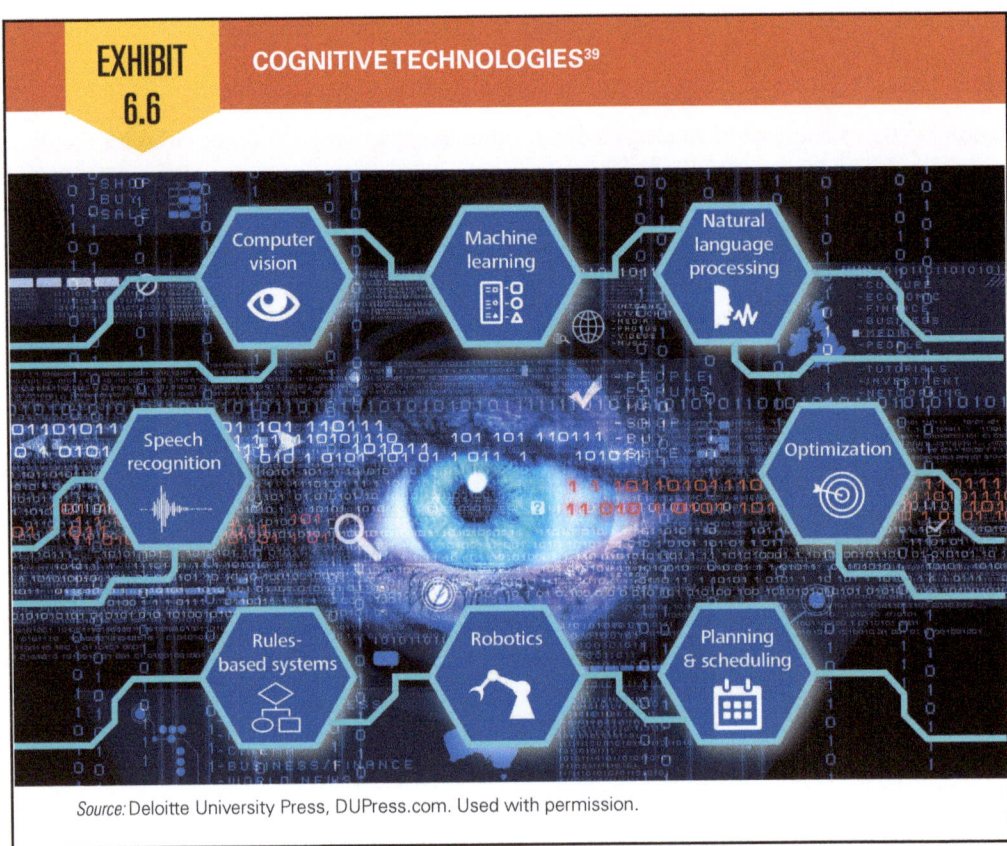

Source: Deloitte University Press, DUPress.com. Used with permission.

According to the Cognitive Computing Consortium, cognitive computing is a new kind of technology processing that "handles human kinds of problems."[42,43] These systems synthesize information based on context, new data, and conflicting evidence and have the ability to think through problems and solutions. To be considered a cognitive tool, a system must demonstrate the following capabilities:

CAPABILITY	REQUIRED FEATURES
Adaptive	A system capable of learning based on new information/inputs.
	Can deal with ambiguity and resolve conflicts.
	Can process real-time or near real-time data.
Interactive	Easy user interface and inputs.
	Interacts with people, devices, and other cloud services.
Iterative and Stateful	Asks questions or delves into alternative sources of information to help define a problem.
	Can remember previous processed interactions and deliver specific information relevant to the problem/application.
Contextual	Can understand, identify, and extract contextual inputs.
	Can use both structured and unstructured digital information.

Source: Cognitive Computing Consortium.com

As you reflect on the cognitive capabilities list you will see that capabilities applied to cognitive computing also apply to artificial intelligence systems.

RESOURCES: AI APPLICATIONS IN USE TODAY

Nursing and AI: Robert, N. (2019). How artificial intelligence is changing nursing. *Journal of Nursing Management*. https://journals.lww.com/nursingmanagement/Fulltext/2019/09000/How_artificial_intelligence_is_changing_nursing.8.aspx

Medical AI Review: Topol, E. J. (2019). High-performance medicine: The convergence of human and artificial intelligence. *Nature Medicine*, 25(1), 44–56.

Robots: Greshko, M. (2018, May 18). Meet Sophia, the robot that looks almost human. *National Geographic*. Retrieved from https://www.nationalgeographic.com/photography/proof/2018/05/sophia-robot-artificial-intelligence-science/

HOW DO COMPUTERS LEARN?

Each AI technology uses combinations of unique algorithms to process data and to generate outputs. Algorithms are automated instructions that tell a computer what to do with the data. The instructions are mathematically driven and can involve multiple layers of mathematical computations. The algorithms can manipulate data in a variety of ways such as sorting, inserting, replacing, or searching for attributes in the data set. The goal for the algorithm is to solve a problem based on mathematical processing. How a machine corrects itself depends on the algorithms selected for the task.

The learning that takes place is captured in algorithms that update based on new data presented. In order for AI systems to learn and update independently of any coded instructions, the system must have massive data sets that are specific to the problem being addressed, and the data must be "clean" so erroneous or biased data has been eliminated. To gain context, in 2011 Andrew Ng, while working at Google, proved that computers could learn. Using 10 million online videos of cats, he successfully trained a computer system to learn what a cat was—this was a technology breakthrough for AI computing. To achieve this goal, the computer system required massive amounts of data, which means that for AI projects you need large data sets *and* the capacity to process them.

Today, *machine learning* is a term often discussed among technology and business teams. Machine learning is a type of AI technology that processes large data sets to solve specific problems. Let's take a look at how a computer can learn.

<table>
<tr><td>

EXERCISE 6.2
</td><td>

FIVE-MINUTE KNOWLEDGE TIDBIT — EXPLORE HOW MACHINES LEARN[44,45]
</td></tr>
</table>

What is machine learning? Provided by MathWorks.com.

Go to https://www.mathworks.com/videos/what-is-machine-learning–1539283415002.html.

Select the video "What is Machine Learning?" by MATLAB (October 17, 2018).

Watch the four-minute video and explore the links on the page to gain an understanding of how machines use data.

<table>
<tr><td>

EXHIBIT 6.7
</td><td>

MACHINE LEARNING
</td></tr>
</table>

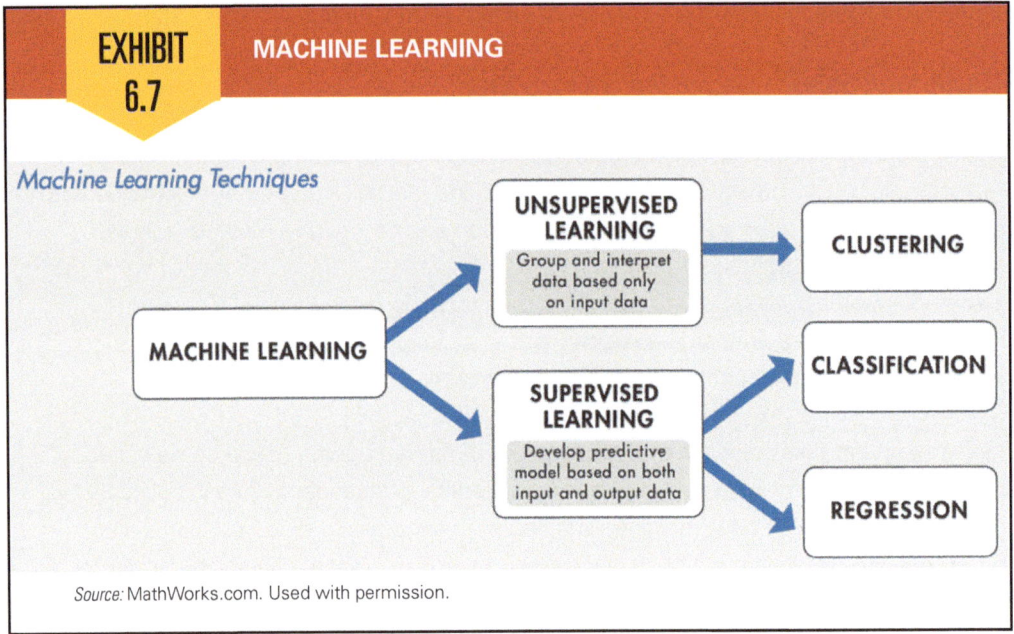

Machine Learning Techniques

Source: MathWorks.com. Used with permission.

If you find yourself working on an AI team you may encounter terms *supervised* and *unsupervised learning* to describe technology used for your project. *Supervised learning* describes a system whereby the computer is trained by providing data inputs that map to a specific data output—this is referred to as a pair of labeled data. Using predefined labeled training data pairs, a computer algorithm is created to examine new data encountered by the system. The system determines whether newly encountered data meets the criteria

EXHIBIT 6.8

SCREENSHOT OF THE JVION MACHINE PORTAL THAT HIGHLIGHTS THE HEALTH REGRESSION VECTOR OUTPUTS

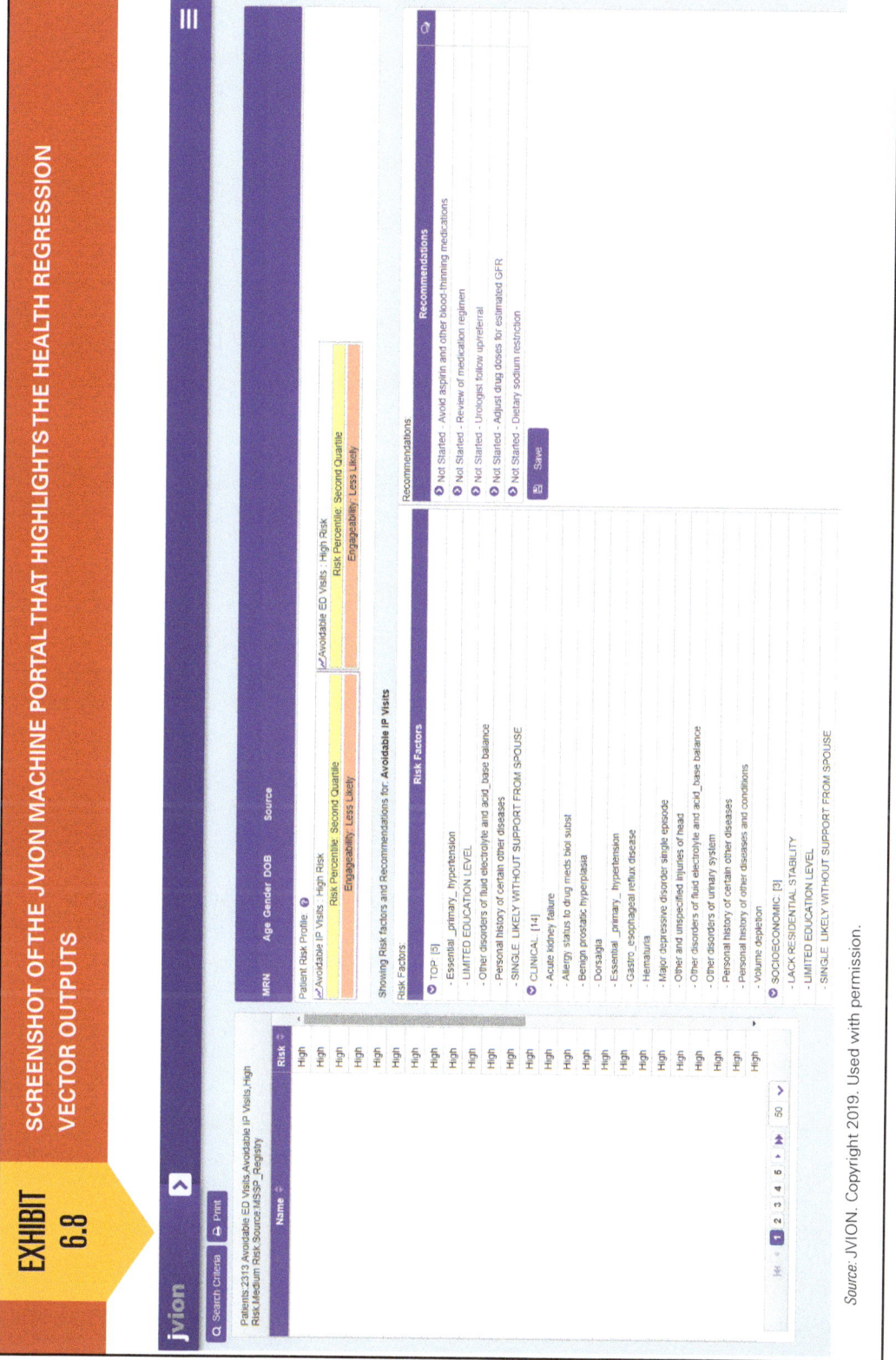

Source: JVION. Copyright 2019. Used with permission.

used to train the system. If the system is trained correctly using input-output data pairs, as new data is encountered the computer will correctly analyze the data and provide results that are accurate. If the training data is not accurate, the old adage "garbage in, garbage out" applies. The data underpins the accuracy of the algorithms and the final results.

Unsupervised learning is a condition where a computer is given large amounts of data with no preconceived notion about what insights or inferences will be found in the data. The computer looks for patterns in data and the data do not have assigned labels. Common outputs from this type of learning are cluster analysis used in exploratory data analysis and association analysis. Using statistical algorithms to process the unlabeled data, the data speaks for itself without any preconceived notion of what the end result will be. The system learns from the data provided, generating insights based on data inputs. Comparatively, supervised data learning systems have an expected outcome based on how the data input mapped to established criteria that determines results presented by the system.

There are significant differences in AI outputs based on data collected, how data is processed within an application, and what objectives the system is trying to achieve. Let's look at two examples of systems in use today.

JVION's *Prescriptive Analytics for Preventable Harm* system is an example of a complex AI system. The AI-eigen based system is designed to process thousands of variables, with a goal to assess health care risks unique to each patient. The system collects data based on hospital encounters, external data sources such as government census data, and third-party data sources that have been carefully vetted to ensure data quality. The AI application follows the patient from the hospital through discharge to home. The algorithms, data inputs and outputs are unique to the AI application, formulating customized profiles to assess risks for each patient.

The Jvion Machine portal requires a health care practitioner to embrace a new orientation of health care analytics based on data collected within hospital systems and data gathered outside of healthcare delivery systems. With thousands of variables being considered to ascertain the status of a patient while in the hospital and upon the patient's discharge to home, the system processes data that health care teams can consider to prevent harm to patients.

A look at a different application, The Rothman Index (RI), targets acuity status *during* a patient's hospital encounter. The RI goal is to identify at-risk patients before they have a critical episode while in the hospital. The RI is based on 26 indicators, with the RI acuity scores generated from data collected from the electronic health record. The RI produces real-time patient acuity scores based on vital signs, laboratory values, and nursing assessments. Eleven of the 26 indicators are based on nursing assessment data. The index has been validated with more than 50 peer-reviewed studies and has been associated with reductions in mortality.[46]

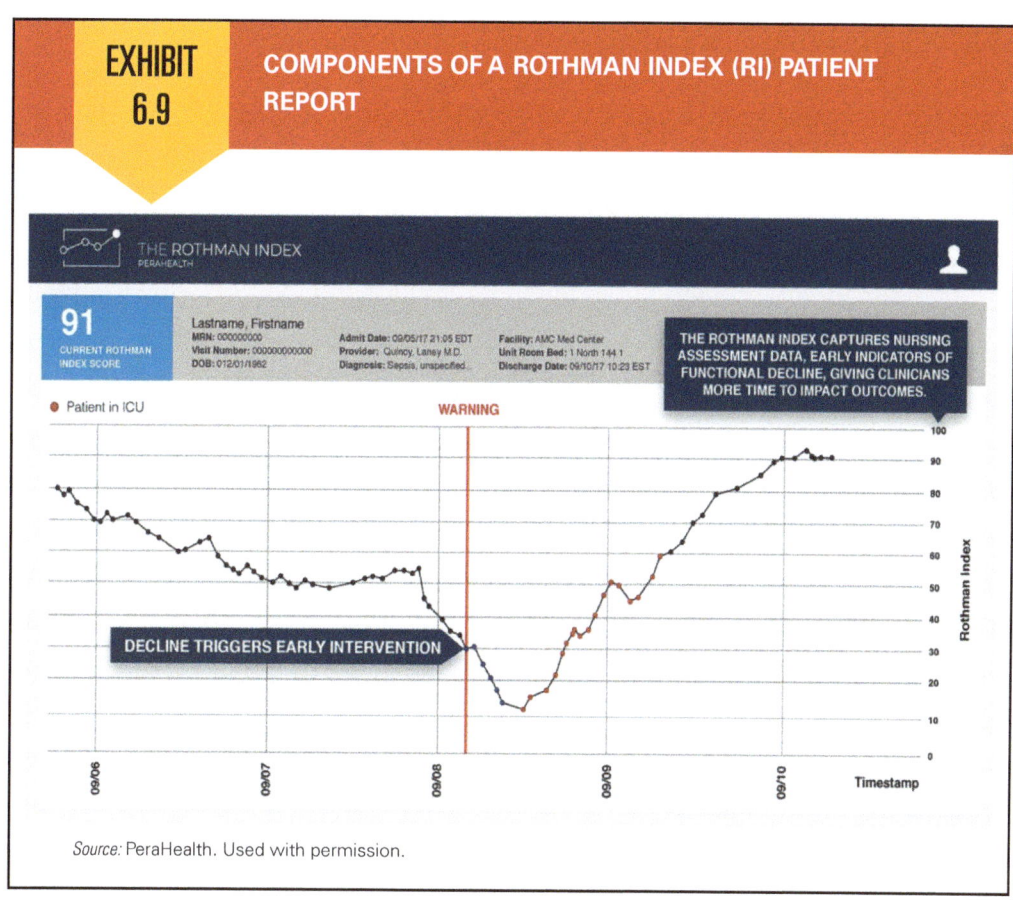

Source: PeraHealth. Used with permission.

Dr. Michael Rothman, co-founder of the RI application, maintains that "There is only one meaningful test for an early warning system, and that is the extent to which it adds incremental value to the delivery of care in the hospital."

Each AI technology has its unique algorithms, mathematical approaches, and data inputs that drive decision outputs and functions performed by health care teams. AI teams are composed of specialists who are trained in specific AI and big data technologies. Machine engineers and data scientists are the experts that create the algorithms and data parameters required to process data. Most healthcare professionals will serve in roles as subject matter experts to address specific questions related to the problem of interest.

Given the pace and volume of new AI and big data systems entering the health care market, health care practitioners need to assess competencies required to:

1. Understand and leverage new patient data sources in the delivery of care.

2. Work with interprofessional teams to align health care protocols.

3. Communicate findings to patients and families.

AI AND BIG DATA TEAMS

As a subject matter expert (SME), or as a team member who is working with an AI team, it is likely that you will be involved in identifying the problem being addressed, will contribute knowledge about key attributes required to analyze the problem, and will be asked to verify the computer results when computer training data and final data results are available. There are many roles on AI and big data teams.

In AI, there are many roles that are frequently mentioned, but the industry does not consistently apply the same role definition across job titles and responsibilities. In general, you may find yourself working with one or more Software Engineers, Machine Learning Engineers who specialize in supervised learning and neural networks, Machine Learning Researchers, Robotics and Vision Engineers, Data Scientists who interpret the data, Data Engineers who organize the data, AI product managers who help identify what is impactful, relevant, and feasible, and SMEs.

TEAM RESOURCES

Big Data Team Level Competency Grid with Performance Indicators created by the United Nations Economic Commission for Europe (UNECE), 2015. The grid provides an overview of team competencies needed to support AI and big data initiatives. Available at: https://www.unece.org/fileadmin /DAM/stats/documents/ece/ces/ge.54/2016/Big_Data_Team _Leader_Nov_2015.pdf

For your convenience a copy of the Big Data Team Level Competency Grid is included in Step 7: Tools and Resources. (See page 211.)

Assess Your Competencies to Work with Big Data and AI

Access the Self-Assessment Critical Thinking Grid in Step 7: Tools and Resources (see page 215). Using the examples in Exhibits 6.8 and 6.9 as a point of reference, reflect on your self-assessment answers regarding your capabilities to integrate data into your professional practice.

CONCLUSION

The world of health care is on a rapid pace of transformation aimed to provide better care, healthy people in healthy communities, and affordable care to all. AI and big data offer the promise of better insights through different thinking. As you learned in Step 5: Innovation, significant investments are being made in AI and cognitive computing systems, and these system investments are expected to continue to impact healthcare. Companies like Amazon are creating new AI-driven programs that leverage natural language programming and deep learning expertise to create HIPAA-eligible products for Amazon Transcription and Comprehend Medical, a medical extraction application that can assess unstructured data from medical notes.[47] Microsoft has entered the clinical cancer space, teaming with scientists and researchers to combat cancer using machine learning and natural language processing.[48] Apple has turned your watch into a "proactive health monitor" that can track your heart readings, manage your fitness and wellness routines, and provide assistance if you fall.[49.] The world of healthcare is rapidly changing, and you can expect that during your career you will be exposed to these technologies and may even find yourself becoming part of an AI or big data team.

RECOMMENDED RESOURCES FOR FURTHER STUDY

If you are interested in gaining a more comprehensive under-standing of AI and its potential access:

- Visit Coursera.org and sign up for Andrew Ng's AI for Everyone course.

- Explore your local university for introductory AI course options.

- Access IBM's Cognitive Computing site and test-drive free tools and educational offerings.

- Access the Deloitte Analytics site and learn about applied AI applications.

REFERENCES

1. Statista Digital Population Worldwide. Retrieved from https://www.statista.com/statistics/617136/digital-population-worldwide/

2. "Smartphone Ownership Is Growing Rapidly Around the World, but Not Always Equally." PEW Research Center, Washington, D.C. (February 5, 2019). Retrieved from https://www.pewresearch.org/global/2019/02/05/smartphone-ownership-is-growing-rapidly-around-the-world-but-not-always-equally/

3. "Internet/Broadband Fact Sheet." PEW Research Center, Washington, D.C. (June 12, 2019). Retrieved from http://www.pewinternet.org/fact-sheet/internet-broadband

4. Paul Hitlin. "Internet, Social Media Use and Device Ownership in U.S. Have Plateaued After Years of Growth." PEW Research Center, Washington, D.C. (September 28, 2018). Retrieved from https://www .pewresearch.org/fact-tank/2018/09/28/internet-social-media-use-and-device-ownership-in-u-s-have -plateaued-after-years-of-growth/

5. Jingjing, Jiang. "Millennials Stand Out for their Technology Use, But Older Generations Also Embrace Digital Life." PEW Research Center, Washington, D.C. (May 2, 2018). Retrieved from http://www .pewinternet.org/fact-tank/2018/05/02/millennials-stand-out-for-their-technology-use-but-older -generations-also-embrace-digital-life/

6. Deloitte. 2019 Global Life Sciences Outlook . Retrieved from https://www2.deloitte.com/global/en /pages/life-sciences-and-healthcare/articles/global-life-sciences-sector-outlook.html.

7. Meeker, M. Internet trends 2018. Kleiner perkins report. Retrieved from https://www.kleinerperkins .com/files/INTERNET_TRENDS_REPORT_2018.pdf

8. Internet of Things connected devices installed base worldwide from 2015 to 2025 (in billions). Retrieved from https://www.statista.com/statistics/471264/iot-number-of-connected-devices-worldwide/

9. DBS Asian Insights, Internet of Things The Pillar of Artificial Intelligence, June 28, 2018 (PDF, 64 pp., no opt-in) https://bigdata-iot.org/2018/12/21/2018-roundup-of-internet-of-things-forecasts-and-market -estimates/

10. Grand View Research, IoT in Healthcare Market Worth $534.3 Billion by 2025, March 2019. Retrieved from https://www.grandviewresearch.com/press-release/global-iot-in-healthcare-market

11. Greg Reh, Eight IoT Barriers for Connected Medical Devices and how to overcome them. Retrieved from https://deloitte.wsj.com/cfo/2018/08/14/eight-iot-barriers-for-connected-medical-devicesand-how-to -overcome-them/

12. Abrams, K. and Korba, C. (2018). Consumers are on board with virtual health options. Can the health system deliver? Deloitte Center for Health Solutions. Retrieved from https://www2.deloitte.com /insights/us/en/multimedia/infographics/virtual-health-care-survey-infographic.html?id=us:2em:3na :4di4630:5awa:6di:MMDDYY:&pkid=1005421. Full 2018 report accessed at: https://www2.deloitte.com /insights/us/en/industry/health-care/virtual-health-care-consumer-experience-survey.html?id=us:2el:3dc :4di4631:5awa:6di:&pkid=1005422

13. Kennith Corbin. "How CIOs Can Prepare for the Healthcare 'Data Tsunami'". CIO. (December 16, 2014). https://www.cio.com/article/2860072/how-cios-can-prepare-for-healthcare-data-tsunami.html

14. Desjardins, J. (2018, July 26). How Big Data Will Unlock the Potential of Health Care. *VisualCapitalist*. Retrieved from https://www.visualcapitalist.com/big-data-healthcare/

15. Dutcher, J. (2014, September 3).What is big data? *Datascience Berkeley edu blog*. Retrieved from http:// datascience.berkeley.edu/what-is-big-data/

16. Marr, B. (2015, March 23). Big data explained in less than 2 minutes. Bernard Marr Blog. Retrieved from https://www.linkedin.com/pulse/big-data-explained-less-than-2-minutes-absolutely-anyone-bernard-marr /trk=mp-reader-card

17. Finos, R. (2016). 2016-2026 Worldwide Big Data Market Forecast. *Wikibon*. Retrieved from http://wikibon .com/2016-2026 -worldwide-big-data-market-forecast/

18. Marr, B. (2015, April 21). How big data is changing healthcare. *Forbes*. Retrieved from http://www.forbes.com/sites/bernardmarr/2015/04/21/how-big-data-is-changing-healthcare/

19. Reichert, J. & Furlong, G. (2014). Five key pillars of an analytics center of excellence, which are required to manage populations and transform organizations into the next era of health care. *Nursing Administration Quarterly, 38*(2):159–165.

20. Marr, B. (2015). Apple and IBM team up for new big data health platform. *LinkedIn*. Retrieved from https://www.linkedin.com/pulse/apple-ibm-team-up-new-big-data-health-platform-bernard-marr

21. Apple Insider. (March 19, 2018). Apple, IBM Partnership Expands With New Machine Learning Integrations. Retrieved from https://appleinsider.com/articles/18/03/20/apple-ibm-partnership-expands-with-new-machine-learning-integrations

22. Pittsburg Health Data Alliance. (2019) Three Pittsburg Institutions. One Goal. Retrieved from http://healthdataalliance.com/

23. Deloitte Development LLC. (2015). *ConvergeHEALTH by Deloitte.* Deloitte University Press. Retrieved from http://www.converge-health.com/ . See https://ww2.deloitte.com/us/en/pages/consulting/topics/convergehealth.html for current projects.

24. National Institute of Health (2014). *NIH Big Data to Knowledge (BD2K) Grants Research and Resource Support.* Retrieved from https://www.nlm.nih.gov/ep/BD2KGrants.html

25. National Institute of Health (2019). *Research Funding.* Retrieved from https://datascience.nih.gov/foa

26. Gens, F. (2014, December). IDC predictions 2015: Accelerating innovation—and growth—on the 3rd platform. *IDC Report.* Retrieved from http://www.idc.com/research/Predictions15/index.jsp;jsessionid=7A245DEABEC9C39AA8C58EABE22DBBF4

27. Petrov, C. (2019, March 22). Big data statistics 2019. TechJury Blog. Retrieved https://techjury.net/stats-about/big-data-statistics/

28. Marr, B. (2014, September 25). Big data: The eye-opening facts everyone should know. Bernard Marr Blog. Retrieved from https://bigdata-madesimple.com/eye-opening-facts-everyone-should-know-about-big-data/

29. McCarthy, M. (2019, May 6. National Nurses Week 2019: Nurses Leading Change in Digital Health Solutions. Microsoft Industry Blogs. Retrieved from https://cloudblogs.microsoft.com/industry-blog/health/2019/05/06/national-nurses-week-2019-nurses-leading-change-in-digital-health-solutions/

30. The Rothman Index. (n.d.). Retrieved from https://www.perahealth.com/the-rothman-index/model-development-and-scientific-validation/

31. Duncan-Finlay, G., Rothman, M.J., & Smith, R.A. (February 2014). Measuring the modified early warning score and the Rothman Index: Advantages of utilizing the electronic medical record in an early warning system. Journal of Hospital Medicine,9. Retrieved from https://www.ncbi.nlm.nih.gov/pmc/articles/PMC4321057/

32. Bates, D.W., Saria, S., Ohno-Machado, L., Shah, A., & Escobar, G. (2014). Big data in health care: Using analytics to identify and manage high-risk and high-cost patients. *Health Affairs, 33*(7):1123–1131.

33. GNS Healthcare. (2014). *AJMC publishes results showing big data analytics can predict risk of metabolic syndrome.* Retrieved from http://www.gnshealthcare.com/ajmc-publishes-results-showing-big-data-analytics-can-predict-risk-of-metabolic-syndrome/

34. Halamka, J.D. (2014). Early experiences with big data at an academic medical center. *Health Affairs*, *33*(7):1132–1138.

35. Howie, L., Hirsch, B., Locklear, T., & Abernethy, A.P. (2014). Assessing the value of patient-generated data to comparative effectiveness research. *Health Affairs, 33*(7):1220–1228.

36. Fihn, S. D., Francis, J., Clancy, C., Nielson, C., Nelson, K., Rumsfeld, J., Cullen, T., Bates, J. & Graham, G. L. (2014). Insights from advanced analytics at the veteran's health administration. *Health Affairs, 33*(7):1203–1211.

37. Krumholz, H. M. (2014). Big data and new knowledge in medicine: The thinking training, and tools needed for a learning health system. *Health Affairs, 33*(7):1163–1170.

38. Roski, J., Bo-Linn, G. W., Andrews, T. A. (2014). Creating value in healthcare through big data: Opportunities and policy implications. *Health Affairs, 33*(7):1115–1122.

39. Deloitte. Demystifying artificial intelligence: What business leaders need to know about cognitive technologies .Retrieved from https://www2.deloitte.com/insights/us/en/focus/cognitive-technologies/what-is -cognitive-technology.html and https://healthitanalytics.com/news/big-data-to-see-explosive-growth -challenging-healthcare-organizations

40. Colom, R., Karama, S., Jung, R. E., & Haier, R. J. (2010). Human intelligence and brain networks. *Dialogues in clinical neuroscience, 12*(4), 489-501.

41. Davenport, T.H., Loucks, J.. & Schatsky. (2017). The Deloitte State of Cognitive Survey. Accessed at https://www2.deloitte.com/content/dam/Deloitte/us/Documents/deloitte-analytics/us-da-2017-deloitte -state-of-cognitive-survey.pdf

42. Cognitive Computing Consortium. Cognitive Computing Definition. Access at https://cognitivecomputing consortium.com/definition-of-cognitive-computing/

43. Cognitive Computing Definition. Accessed at https://cognitivecomputingconsortium.com/definition -of-cognitive-computing/

44. Introducing Machine Learning. Mathworks. Accessed at https://www.mathworks.com/content/dam /mathworks/tag-team/Objects/i/88174_92991v00_machine_learning_section1_ebook.pdf

45. Shure, L. What is Machine Learning? Video. Accessed at https://www.mathworks.com/videos/what -is-machine-learning--1539283415002.html

46. Walsh, K., Hamlin, S., & Askary, B. (2016). Mortality reduction associated with surveillance using an emr-based acuity score at an academic medical center. *BMJ Quality & Safety*, 25, 1014-1015.

47. Amazon Comprehend Medical. Retrieved at https://aws.amazon.com/comprehend/medical/

48. Linn, A. How Microsoft computer scientists and researchers are working to 'solve' cancer, https://news .microsoft.com/stories/computingcancer/

49. Apple Watch Series 4, https://www.apple.com/apple-watch-series-4/health/

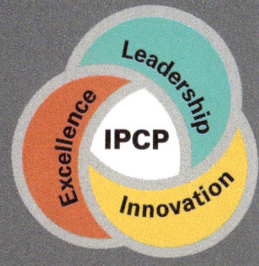

TOOLS AND RESOURCES

FUNDAMENTALS OF MAGNET®
GAP ANALYSIS TOOL

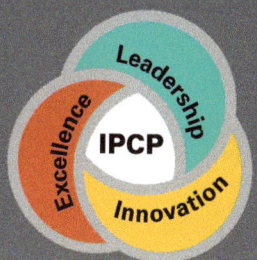

Connecting Magnet® Recognition to ACA Outcomes

Nursing strategies align with organizational priorities that include quality, safety, patient-centered care, prevention, and affordability.

YES   NO

The chief nursing officer (CNO) influences organizational change and strategic decisions that impact organizational strategies and tactics outside of nursing.

YES   NO

Nursing participation is an essential component of interprofessional decision-making in the organization.

YES   NO

Organizational resources are provided to support nursing in the delivery of education to patients and families.

YES   NO

Nursing is involved in identifying community healthcare needs.

YES   NO

Nurses provide patient-centered care through the development and use of individualized care plans.

YES   NO

Nurses are members of interprofessional collaborative teams for coordination and continuity of patient care.

YES   NO

National patient safety goals are considered in the evaluation of clinical practice.

YES   NO

The organization has a method to collect patient satisfaction and nurse-sensitive clinical data at the unit level, and the data is benchmarked.

YES   NO

Nurses use evidence-based decision-making processes to guide clinical practice.

YES   NO

Resources are in place to disseminate new knowledge and innovations in support of nursing practice.

YES   NO

Evaluate gaps

Consider application for Magnet

173

Connecting Magnet® Recognition to ACA Outcomes

Nursing strategies align with organizational priorities that include quality, safety, patient-centered care, prevention, and affordability.	NO	Evaluate gap

YES

	YES	NO
Are organizational strategies aligned with improving the overall quality of care by making health care more patient-centered, reliable, accessible, and safe?	☐	☐
Are nursing's mission, vision, values, and strategic plan aligned with the organization's priorities to improve the organization's performance? (TL1EO)	☐	☐
Do nurse leaders and clinical nurses advocate for resources to support nursing unit and organizational goals? (TL2)	☐	☐
Are nurses recognized for their contributions in addressing the strategic priorities of the organization? (SE11)	☐	☐

NOTES

_____
_____
_____
_____

The chief nursing officer (CNO) influences organizational change and strategic decisions that impact organizational strategies and tactics outside of nursing.	NO	Evaluate gap

YES

	YES	NO
Is there evidence that the CNO is a peer of the organization's C-suite executives who drive the delivery of effective, patient-family centered, reliable, accessible, safe, and affordable care?	☐	☐
Does the CNO influence organization-wide change beyond the scope of nursing? (TL3EO)	☐	☐
Does the CNO serve as a strategic partner in the organization's decision-making? (TL4)	☐	☐

NOTES

_____
_____
_____
_____

Connecting Magnet® Recognition to ACA Outcomes

Nursing participation is an essential component of interprofessional decision-making in the organization.	NO	Evaluate gap
YES		

	YES	NO
Does the organization bring together health professions to foster high-performing interprofessional teams and patient care models that promote the delivery of better care?	☐	☐
Are clinical nurses involved in interprofessional decision-making groups in the organization? (SE1EO)	☐	☐
Do nurses assume leadership roles (leader or coleader) in interprofessional activities that improve the quality of care? (EP12)	☐	☐
Are nurses involved in the organization's approach and focused on proactive risk assessment and error management? (EP19EO)	☐	☐

NOTES

_____

_____

_____

_____

Organizational resources are provided to support nursing in the delivery of education to patients and families.	NO	Evaluate gap
YES		

	YES	NO
Does the organization promote effective communication and care coordination?	☐	☐
Does the organization engage patients and families in treatment decisions?	☐	☐
Does the organization provide opportunities to improve nurses' expertise to effectively teach patients and families? (SE6)	☐	☐
Do nurses participate in interprofessional groups that implement and evaluate coordinated patient education activities? (EP13EO)	☐	☐

NOTES

_____

_____

_____

_____

Connecting Magnet® Recognition to ACA Outcomes

Nursing is involved in identifying community healthcare needs.	NO Evaluate gap

YES

	YES	NO
Does the organization work with communities to promote wide use of best practices to enable healthy living?	☐	☐
Do nurses participate in the assessment and prioritization of the healthcare needs of the community? (SE10EO)	☐	☐
Does the organization support nurses' participation in community healthcare outreach? (SE9)	☐	☐

NOTES

_____
_____
_____
_____

Nurses provide patient-centered care through the development and use of individualized care plans.	NO Evaluate gap

YES

	YES	NO
Do patients receive individualized transition care plans upon discharge? (See CTM-3 measures for examples of transition care information.)	☐	☐
Do nurses create partnerships with patients and families to establish goals and plans for delivery of patient-centered care? (EP4)	☐	☐

NOTES

_____
_____
_____
_____

Connecting Magnet® Recognition to ACA Outcomes

Nurses are members of interprofessional collaborative teams for coordination and continuity of patient care.

YES   **NO**   **Evaluate gap**

	YES	NO
Does the organization promote effective communication and coordination of patient care by engaging a healthcare team that optimizes physician, nursing, and other healthcare provider contributions, as allowed by governing regulatory bodies, to provide integrated patient care?	☐	☐
Are nursing quality and patient safety plans, patient policies (privacy, security, confidentiality, patient ethics, and nondiscrimination), and nursing practices integrated with interprofessional patient care decisions in the organization?	☐	☐
Do nurse leaders, with clinical nurse input, use trended data to acquire necessary resources to support the care delivery system(s)? (TL7)	☐	☐
Are nurses involved in interprofessional collaborative practice to ensure care coordination and continuity of care? (EP5)	☐	☐
Is nurse autonomy supported and promoted through the organization's governance structure for shared decision-making? (EP16)	☐	☐

NOTES

_____

_____

_____

_____

Connecting Magnet® Recognition to ACA Outcomes

National patient safety goals are considered in the evaluation of clinical practice.	NO	Evaluate gap

YES

	YES	NO
Does the organization have processes in place to make care safer by reducing harm caused in the delivery of care?	☐	☐
Does the nursing patient safety plan incorporate national and international patient safety goals into requirements for nursing practice? (EP21EO)	☐	☐
Are clinical nurses involved in the review, action planning, and evaluation of patient safety data at the unit level? (EP20EO)	☐	☐

NOTES

_____

_____

_____

_____

The organization has a method to collect patient satisfaction and nurse-sensitive clinical data at the unit level, and the data is benchmarked.	NO	Evaluate gap

YES

	YES	NO
Does the organization provide patient-reported experience and data measures at the unit or clinic level?	☐	☐
Does the unit- or clinic-level patient-satisfaction data (nursing related) outperform the mean or median of a national database? (EP23EO)	☐	☐
Does the unit- or clinic-level nurse-sensitive clinical data outperform the mean or median of a national database? (EP22EO)	☐	☐

NOTES

_____

_____

_____

_____

Connecting Magnet® Recognition to ACA Outcomes

Nurses use evidence based decision-making processes to guide clinical practice.	NO	Evaluate gap
YES		

	YES	NO
The IOM Roundtable on Value and Science-Driven Health Care expects 90% of healthcare decisions in the United States to be evidence-based by 2020. Does the organization have structures and processes to integrate evidence into patient decisions?	☐	☐
Do clinical nurses evaluate and use evidence-based findings in their clinical practice? (NK3)	☐	☐
Are resources, such as professional literature, readily available to support decision-making in autonomous nursing practice? (EP14)	☐	☐

NOTES

_____
_____
_____
_____

Resources are in place to disseminate new knowledge and innovations in support of nursing practice.	NO	Evaluate gap
YES		

	YES	NO
Are nurses included in the design and implementation of workflow and space design improvements and nursing innovations that impact the delivery of patient care (safety, coordination, prevention, treatment, cost) in the organization?	☐	☐
Is the CNO a strategic partner in the organization's technology decision-making? (TL4)	☐	☐
Are clinical nurses involved with the design and implementation of technology to enhance the patient experience and nursing practice? (NK5EO)	☐	☐
Do clinical nurses have the structure and process in place to evaluate and use evidence-based findings? (NK3)	☐	☐

NOTES

_____
_____
_____
_____

ACCREDITATION CROSSWALK

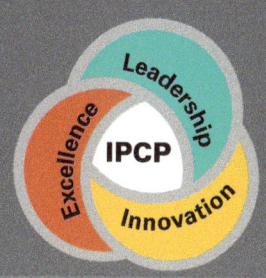

	ANCC	ACCME	ACPE	JOINT ACCREDITATION
Mission statement and goals	The provider is required to identify quality outcome measures it collects, evaluates, and monitors specific to the Provider Unit and to Nursing Professional Development. A written mission statement is not required.	The provider has a CME mission statement that includes expected results articulated in terms of changes in competence, performance, or patient outcomes that will be the result of the program.	The provider has a CPE goal and mission statement that defines the basis and intended outcomes for the majority of educational activities. The CPE mission statement is consistent with the goals, indicates the provider's short-term intent in conducting CPE activities, includes the intended audience, and includes the scope of activities.	The accredited provider has a continuing education (CE) mission statement that highlights education for the healthcare team as part of their purpose, content areas, target audience, type of activities, and expected results, with the expected results articulated in terms of changes in skills/strategy, or performance of the healthcare team or in patient outcomes.
Goals and quality outcome measures related to the overall program of CE	The provider is required to identify quality outcome measures it collects, evaluates, and monitors specific to the Provider Unit and to Nursing Professional Development.	The provider gathers data or information and conducts a program-based analysis on the degree to which the CME mission of the provider has been met through the conduct of CME activities/educational interventions. The provider identifies, plans, and implements the needed or desired changes in the overall program (e.g., planners, teachers, infrastructure, methods, resources, facilities, interventions) that are required to improve on ability to meet the CME mission.	The provider assesses achievement and impact of stated mission and goals. The provider has an evaluation plan that includes collecting data and analyzing it to document achievement of the mission and goals. The provider uses assessment information for continuous development and improvement of the CPE program.	The provider gathers data or information and conducts a program-based analysis on the degree to which the CE mission of the provider has been met through the conduct of CE activities/educational interventions.
Integration of Continuing Education for the Healthcare Team				The provider operates in a manner that integrates CE into the process for improving the professional practice of the healthcare team.
Assessment of learner needs	The provider assesses learner needs (knowledge, skill/competence, practice/performance) that contribute to the professional practice gap and has supporting data to validate the need for the educational activity.	The provider incorporates into CME activities the educational needs (knowledge, competence, or performance) that underlie the professional practice gaps of their own learners.	The provider includes the identification of educational needs as one of the several procedures for developing CPE activities.	The provider incorporates into CE activities the educational needs (knowledge, skills/strategy, or performance) that underlie the practice gaps of the healthcare team and/or the individual members of the healthcare team.

	ANCC	ACCME	ACPE	JOINT ACCREDITATION
Professional practice gap	The provider identifies a professional practice gap for registered nurses that may include but is not limited to a change that has been made to a standard of care, a problem that exists in practice, or an opportunity for improvement.	The provider incorporates into CME activities the educational needs (knowledge, competence, or performance) that underlie the professional practice gaps of their own learners.	Needs assessments employ multiple strategies to identify the specific gaps in knowledge, skills, and/or practice.	The provider incorporates into CE activities the educational needs (knowledge, skills/strategy, or performance) that underlie the practice gaps of the healthcare team and/or the individual members of the healthcare team.
Planning Committee	The Planning Committee must include one nurse prepared at baccalaureate level or higher (Nurse Planner) and one other person; one individual must have content expertise in subject area.		The planning committee (if applicable) should include members of the target audience.	Planners must be representative of the target audience.
Roles of planning committee members	The Nurse Planner is responsible for compliance of the educational activity with ANCC accreditation criteria.		Although not required, if a planning committee is used, it should include members of the targeted audience of the CPE activity.	
Evaluation of conflict of interest	The Nurse Planner is responsible for evaluating presence or absence of conflict of interest for each individual in a position to control content of the educational activity (planner, faculty, presenter, author, content reviewer). Identified conflicts must be resolved.	The provider develops activities/educational interventions independent of commercial interests. (SCS 1, 2, and 6).	The provider has policies and procedures to ensure that the planning, implementation, and evaluation of educational activities are done without the influence or control of the commercial interest.	The provider develops activities/educational interventions that are independent of commercial interests (ACCME Standards for Commercial SupportSM), including the: a. Identification, resolution, and disclosure of relevant financial relationships of all individuals who control the content of the continuing education activity; b. Appropriate management of commercial support (if applicable). c. Maintenance of the separation of promotion from education (if applicable). d. Promotion of improvements in health care and NOT proprietary interests of a commercial interest.

	ANCC	ACCME	ACPE	JOINT ACCREDITATION
Purpose of educational activity	The provider identifies the learning outcome(s) participants are expected to achieve as a result of participating in the educational activity.	The provider generates activities/educational interventions that are designed to change competence, performance, or patient outcomes as described in its mission statement.	The educational activity addresses the identified knowledge, skill and/or practice gaps.	The provider generates activities/educational interventions that are designed to change the skills/strategy, performance of the healthcare team, or patient outcomes.
Objectives	Not required.	The provider generates activities/educational interventions that are designed to change competence, performance, or patient outcomes as described in its mission statement.	The provider develops specific and measurable objectives for each CPE activity. The objectives are appropriate for the activity-type selected (Knowledge, Application, or Practice-based) for what a pharmacist and/or pharmacy technician will be able to do at the completion of the activity.	The provider generates activities/educational interventions that are designed to change the skills/strategy, performance of the healthcare team, or patient outcomes.
Applicability of content to learners	Content of the educational activity is congruent with the desired learning outcome(s).	The provider incorporates into CME activities the educational needs (knowledge, competence, or performance) that underlie the professional practice gaps of their own learners.	The provider structures each CPE activity to meet the knowledge-, application, and/or practice-based educational needs of pharmacists and/or pharmacy technicians.	The provider generates activities/educational interventions around valid content that matches the healthcare team's current or potential scope of professional activities.
Content of educational activities	Content is based on current and best-available evidence (evidence-based practice, literature/peer review journals, clinical guidelines, best practices, expert opinion).	1. All the recommendations involving clinical medicine in a CME activity must be based on evidence that is accepted within the profession of medicine as adequate justification for their indications and contraindications in the care of patients. 2. All scientific research referred to, reported, or used in CME in support or justification of a patient care recommendation must conform to the generally accepted standards of experimental design, data collection, and analysis.	The content of the provider's CPE activities is based on evidence as accepted in the literature by the healthcare professions.	The provider generates activities/educational interventions around valid content that matches the healthcare team's current or potential scope of professional activities.

	ANCC	ACCME	ACPE	JOINT ACCREDITATION
Content of educational activities (continued)		3. Providers are not eligible for ACCME accreditation or reaccreditation if they present activities that promote recommendations, treatment, or manners of practicing medicine that are not within the definition of CME, or known to have risks or dangers that outweigh the benefits or known to be ineffective in the treatment of patients. An organization whose program of CME is devoted to advocacy of unscientific modalities of diagnosis or therapy is not eligible to apply for ACCME accreditation.		
Teaching/ educational formats	The provider chooses educational formats for activities/interventions that are appropriate for the setting, objectives, and desired results of the activity. The provider must incorporate ways to actively engage learners in the educational activity. Strategies to engage learners may include but are not limited to integrating opportunities for dialogue or question/answer, including time for self-check or reflection; analyzing case studies; and providing opportunities for problem-based learning.	The provider chooses educational formats for activities/interventions that are appropriate for the setting, objectives, and desired results of the activity.	The provider designs and implements learning activities to foster active participation as a component of live and home study CPE instructional approaches using a variety of techniques including pre- and post-testing, quizzes, case studies, simulation exercises, problem-solving, group discussion, etc.	The provider chooses educational formats for activities/interventions that are appropriate for the setting, objectives, and desired results of the activity.

	ANCC	ACCME	ACPE	JOINT ACCREDITATION
Competencies	No requirement.	The provider develops activities/ educational interventions in the context of desirable physician attributes (e.g., Institute of Medicine (IOM) competencies, or Accreditation Council for Graduate Medical Education (ACGME) Competencies).	The provider develops activities aligned with the competencies required of pharmacists and pharmacy technicians as outlined in: • The JCPP Future Vision of Pharmacy Practice • The AACP, Center for the Advancement of Pharmaceutical Education • The NAPLEX Competency Statements • The PTCB Exam Content Outline	The provider develops activities/ educational interventions in the context of desirable attributes of the healthcare team (e.g., Institute of Medicine competencies, professional competencies, healthcare team competencies, values/ethics, roles and responsibilities, interprofessional communication, teams and teamwork).
Evaluation at the activity level	The provider analyzes changes in learners (knowledge, skill/competence, and/or practice/performance) achieved as a result of participation in the educational activity.	The provider analyzes changes in learners (competence, performance, or patient outcomes) achieved as a result of the overall program's activities/educational interventions.	The provider and faculty include learning assessments in each CPE activity for participants to assess the content learned. Learner feedback is consistent with the objectives and activity type. The provider must have an evaluation process for its CPE activities.	The provider analyzes changes in the healthcare team (skills/strategy, performance, or patient outcomes) achieved as a result of the overall program's activities/educational interventions.
Evaluation at the program level	The provider evaluates its overall program of CE	The provider gathers data or information and conducts a program-based analysis on the degree to which the CME mission of the provider has been met through the conduct of CME activities/educational interventions.	The provider has an evaluation plan that includes collecting data and analyzing it to document achievement of the mission and goals. The provider uses assessment information for continuous development and improvement of the CPE program.	The provider gathers data or information and conducts a program-based analysis on the degree to which the CE mission of the provider has been met through the conduct of CE activities/educational interventions.

	ANCC	ACCME	ACPE	JOINT ACCREDITATION
Contact hour/credit hour	CNE is awarded based on a 60 minute hour; content may be delivered asynchronously; no minimum required	AMA PRA Category 1 credit requirements	ACPE credit is awarded to three types of CPE activities: 1. Knowledge-based CPE activity. These CPE activities are primarily constructed to transmit knowledge (i.e., facts). The minimum amount of credit for these activities is 15 minutes or 0.25 contact hour. 2. Application-based CPE activity. These CPE activities are primarily constructed to apply the information learned in the time frame allotted. The minimum amount of credit for these activities is 60 minutes or one contact hour. 3. Practice-based CPE activity. These CPE activities are primarily constructed to instill, expand, or enhance practice competencies through the systematic achievement of specified knowledge, skills, attitudes, and performance behaviors. The formats of these CPE activities should include a didactic component and a practice experience component. The provider should employ an instructional design that is rationally sequenced, curricular based, and supportive of achievement of the stated professional competencies. The minimum amount of credit for these activities is 15 contact hours.	Continuing education credit awarded for all activities will meet the specific requirements for medicine (AMA PRA Category 1 credit), nursing, and pharmacy.

	ANCC	ACCME	ACPE	JOINT ACCREDITATION
Verification of participation/ successful completion	Learners receive documentation of successful completion of the activity.	An accredited provider must have mechanisms in place to record and, when authorized by the participating physician, verify participation for six years from the date of the CME activity.	As of January 1, 2013, all CPE credit will be uploaded into CPE Monitor™. ACPE and the National Association of Boards of Pharmacy (NABP) developed a continuing pharmacy education (CPE) tracking service, CPE Monitor™, that will authenticate and store data for completed CPE units received by pharmacists and pharmacy technicians from ACPE-accredited providers.	Jointly accredited organizations must have a mechanism in place to verify participation of learners.
Accreditation statement	ANCC accreditation statement must be provided to learners prior to the start of the educational activity and on the certificate of completion "Name of Provider" is accredited as a provider of continuing nursing education by the American Nurses Credentialing Center.	The accreditation statement must appear on all CME activity materials and brochures distributed by accredited organizations, except that the accreditation statement does not need to be included on initial, save-the-date type activity announcements. Such announcements contain only general, preliminary information about the activity such as the date, location, and title. If more specific information is included, such as faculty and objectives, the accreditation statement must be included. The accredited provider must inform the learner of the joint providership relationship through the use of the appropriate accreditation statement. All printed materials for jointly provided activities must carry the appropriate accreditation statement.	Any reference by an accredited provider to accreditation by the Board in announcements, promotional materials, publications, or in any other form of communication or publicity, shall state only the following: "(Name of Provider) is accredited by the Accreditation Council for Pharmacy Education as a provider of continuing pharmacy education." The ACPE logo shall also be used in close conjunction with the statement…	All education materials, marketing materials, certificates, and other documents distributed by the jointly accredited organization that indicate continuing education "credit" will be awarded for completion of the activity, must include the accreditation statement that reflects Joint Accreditation. The accreditation statement to be used is: "[Insert name of Joint Accredited Provider] is accredited by the Accreditation Council for Continuing Medical Education (ACCME), the Accreditation Council for Pharmacy Education (ACPE), and the American Nurses Credentialing Center (ANCC) to provide continuing education for the healthcare team." When an activity has been planned, implemented and evaluated by two or more organizations and one of the organizations has been jointly accredited, the accreditation statement to be used is:

	ANCC	ACCME	ACPE	JOINT ACCREDITATION
Accreditation statement (continued)				"This activity is planned and implemented by [insert name of Joint Accredited Provider and [insert name of other provider]. [Insert name of Joint Accredited Provider] is accredited by the Accreditation Council for Continuing Medical Education (ACCME), the Accreditation Council for Pharmacy Education (ACPE), and the American Nurses Credentialing Center (ANCC) to provide continuing education for the healthcare team." The accreditation must stand alone from any other statement.
Commercial Support	ANCC Content Integrity Standards for Industry Support in Continuing Nursing Educational Activities	The provider appropriately manages commercial support (if applicable, SCS 3 of the ACCME Standards for Commercial SupportSM).	The provider appropriately manages commercial support (if applicable, SCS 3 of the ACCME Standards for Commercial SupportSM).	The provider develops activities/educational interventions that are independent of commercial interests (ACCME Standards for Commercial SupportSM), including the: a. Identification, resolution, and disclosure of relevant financial relationships of all individuals who control the content of the continuing education activity. b. Appropriate management of commercial support (if applicable). c. Maintenance of the separation of promotion from education (if applicable). d. Promotion of improvements in health care and NOT proprietary interests of a commercial interest.

	ANCC	ACCME	ACPE	JOINT ACCREDITATION
Independence from commercial influence	Planning, implementation, and evaluation of educational activities must be independent from the influence of commercial interest organization.	The provider develops activities/ educational interventions independent of commercial interests (SCS 1, 2, and 6).	The provider develops activities/ educational interventions independent of commercial interests (SCS 1, 2, and 6).	The provider develops activities/ educational interventions that are independent of commercial interests (ACCME Standards for Commercial SupportSM), including the: a. Identification, resolution, and disclosure of relevant financial relationships of all individuals who control the content of the continuing education activity. b. Appropriate management of commercial support (if applicable). c. Maintenance of the separation of promotion from education (if applicable). d. Promotion of improvements in health care and NOT proprietary interests of a commercial interest.

	ANCC	ACCME	ACPE	JOINT ACCREDITATION
Required disclosures	The following information must be provided to learners prior to participation in the educational activity. • Presence or absence of COI for any individual having the opportunity to influence the content of an educational activity • Requirements for successful completion of the activity • Commercial support, if applicable • Expiration date, enduring materials only • Joint providership, if applicable	The provider maintains a separation of promotion from education (SCS 4). The provider actively promotes improvements in health care and NOT proprietary interests of a commercial interest (SCS 5).	The provider maintains a separation of promotion from education (SCS 4). The provider actively promotes improvements in health care and NOT proprietary interests of a commercial interest (SCS 5).	The provider develops activities/educational interventions that are independent of commercial interests (ACCME Standards for Commercial Support℠), including the: a. Identification, resolution, and disclosure of relevant financial relationships of all individuals who control the content of the continuing education activity. b. Appropriate management of commercial support (if applicable). c. Maintenance of the separation of promotion from education (if applicable). d. Promotion of improvements in health care and NOT proprietary interests of a commercial interest.
Recordkeeping	Records are kept for 6 years.	An accredited provider must have mechanisms in place to record and, when authorized by the participating physician, verify participation for six years from the date of the CME activity. An accredited provider is required to retain activity files/records of CME activity planning and presentation during the current accreditation term or for the last twelve months, whichever is longer.	The provider shall maintain and assure the availability of records adequate to serve the needs of the learners and others requiring such information for a period of six years. The provider should assure the security of its records by having appropriate backup systems and contingency plans.	The provider maintains and reports required data and information about the continuing education that is delivered during its current term of accreditation. Activity files must be retained by the jointly accredited organization for six years following provision of the educational activity.

	ANCC	ACCME	ACPE	JOINT ACCREDITATION
Joint Providership	ANCC accredited providers that collaborate with ANCC and/or non-ANCC accredited providers are engaging in joint providership. ANCC expects all educational activities to be in compliance with ANCC accreditation requiremetns. It is the accredited provider's responsibility to demonstrate to ANCC compliance through written documentation.	The ACCME expects all CME activities to be in compliance with the accreditation requirements. In cases of joint providership, it is the ACCME accredited provider's responsibility to be able to demonstrate through written documentation this compliance to the ACCME. Materials submitted that demonstrate compliance may be from either the ACCME accredited provider's files or those of the non-accredited provider. The ACCME allows accredited providers and non-accredited organizations (that are not ACCME-defined commercial interests) to collaborate in the planning and implementation of CME activities through joint providership. In joint providership, either the accredited provider or its non-accredited joint provider can control the identification of CME needs, the determination of educational objectives, the selection and presentation of content, the selection of all persons and organizations that will be in a position to control CME content, the selection of educational methods, and the evaluation of the activity.	ACPE accredited providers that collaborate on content development with ACPE and/or non-ACPE accredited providers are engaging in joint providership. ACPE expects all CPE activities to be in compliance with the Accreditation Standards for Continuing Pharmacy Education. It is the accredited provider's responsibility to demonstrate to ACPE compliance through written documentation.	The provider may choose to collaborate with another accredited or non-accredited organization to provide educational activities. The Jointly Accredited Provider is responsible for ensuring that the educational activity is in full compliance with accreditation requirements. The term "Joint Collaboration" will be used to reflect the collaborative relationship between the two organizations (i.e., "This educational activity has been a Joint Collaboration between _____ and _____.")". A Joint Collaboration Agreement is required between the Jointly Accredited Provider and the other accredited or non-accredited organizations. An ACCME-defined commercial interest may not be the collaborating non-accredited organization.
Engagement criteria	Not applicable	Criteria 16–22 are required, in addition to 1–13, if a provider seeks Accreditation with Commendation (6 years).	Not applicable	

TWELVE COMMON LEADERSHIP ACTIVITIES

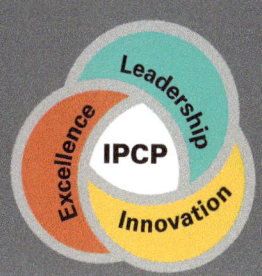

TABLE 1
TWELVE COMMON LEADERSHIP ACTIVITIES

	ACTIVITY	DESCRIPTION
	Team Metrics	Setting team's goals/objectives/KPIs/balanced scorecard and ensuring proper performance tracking mechanisms are in place
	Team Performance Management	This includes regular (daily, weekly, monthly and quarterly) team meetings to review the team's performance against goals and objectives, KPIs, balanced scorecard and making appropriate improvements
	Projects and Initiatives	Identification and the review of initiatives/projects to improve the team's performance (process improvement, customer experience, team member engagement, value creation)
	Plans and Budgets	Development, execution and progress review of the team's operational and workforce plans and budget (this is generally a team's one-year plan and budget with rolling three months forecast)
	Team Sizing and Scheduling Work	Development of team sizing models, work schedules and assignments to meet volume / commitment requirements. (Includes development, implementation, assessment and renewal)
	Staffing	Resourcing the team through the selection of new team members, their on boarding, and development plans. Also managing the team member movement to and from the team.
	Processes and Work Clarity	Ensuring team processes and work ownership clarity exists including clarity of responsibility for outputs, activities, tasks and RACI
	Coaching	Coaching and development of each other on team cultural attributes, norms, member's performance models (critical results and best practices) and over all team leadership skills.

Source: © Gustavson and Liff (2014). Used with permission. From *A Team of Leaders*.

	ACTIVITY	DESCRIPTION
	Team Meetings	Facilitating the team's meetings from developing the agenda, leading the meetings, making sure notes and follow up occur after the meeting while ensuring team participation and ownership of agreements.
	Training and Development	Updating the team on product, policy, process, standards etc. through engaging learning techniques that enhance the team's effectiveness.
	Individual Performance Management	Development and regular review of individual team member's performance and development plans. This includes when necessary dealing with performance problems, establishing performance improvement plans, and making deselection and award recommendations.
	Resource Coordination	Ensures proper coordination with other teams, support groups and partners necessary to complete their work and deliver on the team's commitments

NEW MODEL OF WORK

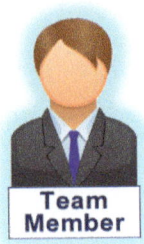
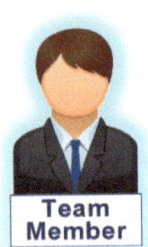
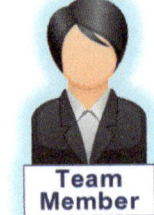
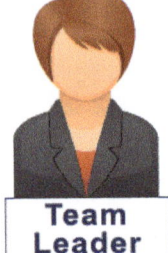
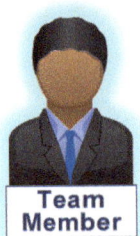

- Leadership is shared

- Knowledge shared

- Team does planning and accountability

- Everyone is highly engaged, involved and motivated

- Leader allowed to do higher level work

- Much better results

Team Member

Team Member

Team Leader

Team Member

Team Member

TABLE 2
FIVE STAGES TO TEAM OF LEADERS

	Stage 1	Primarily one-on-one interaction between the Leader and each team member.
	Stage 2	Leader led with some interaction between team members.
	Stage 3	Leadership begins to be shared as some team members step up and provide leadership while engaging other team members. The team leader assists team members to step up into leadership roles.
	Stage 4	Leadership is shared as most team members are stepping up and providing leadership while engaging with other members. Leader coaches the team to the next level but has time to higher level work.
	Stage 5	Leadership is shared, as all team members are providing leadership, setting and attaining challenging performance targets, benchmarking and establishing best practices and contributing to other teams. The team leader is free to do higher level work outside the team but is still available for counsel.

TEAM OF LEADERS
ASSESSMENT SURVEY

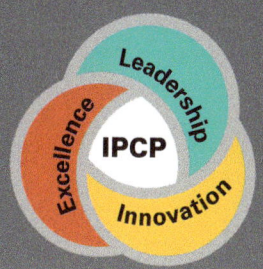

The figure below shows the migration of the role of the formal team leader as the role evolves from being a team leader directing most of the team's activities to an environment where the team owns and performs almost all of the leadership tasks, allowing the team leader to work mostly on higher level tasks. In the following section, please consider each type of work that your team performs, and apportion the percentage of time that the team fits into each of the stages.

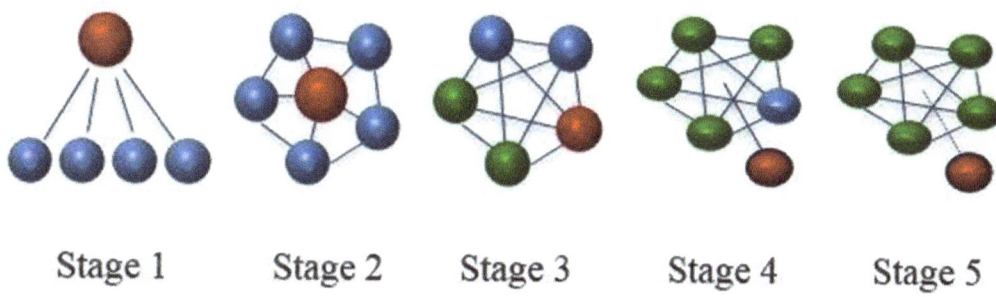

FIGURE 1
STAGES OF TEAM DEVELOPMENT

Source: © Gustavson, Liff & Rhodes (2014). Used with permission. From *A Team of Leaders*.

TEAM OF LEADERS ASSESSMENT SURVEY

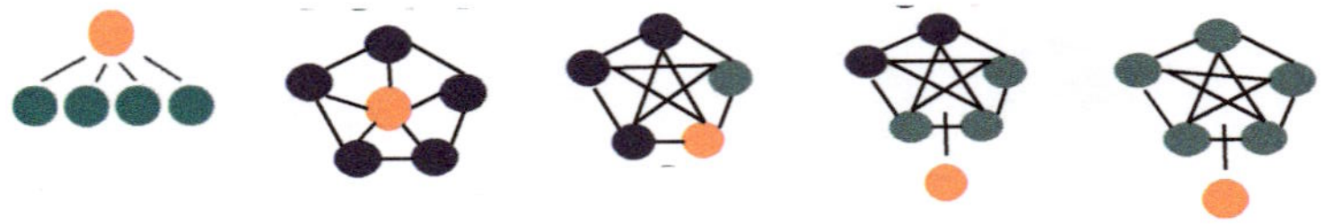

	Primarily performed by the Team Leader through one on ones.	Primarily performed by the team leader in team meeting environments.	Some Team members step up to lead but others depend on the team leader	Leadership is shared where most team members step up to lead. The team leader takes the role of coach and is allowed some time to do higher order work.	Completely a team of leaders. All team members step up to lead—freeing the team leader to do higher order work.
Team Metrics— Setting Team's Goals I Objectives/ KPI's / Balanced Scorecard and ensuring proper performance tracking mechanisms are in place.	☐	☐	☐	☐	☐
Team Performance Management—This includes regular (daily, weekly, monthly & quarterly) team meetings to review the team's performance against goals & objectives, KPI's, balanced scorecard & making appropriate improvements.	☐	☐	☐	☐	☐
Projects and Initiatives—Identification and the review of initiatives/ projects to improve the team's performance (process improvement, customer experience, team member engagement. value creation).	☐	☐	☐	☐	☐
Plans and Budgets— Development, execution and progress review of the team's operational & workforce plans & budget (this is generally a team's one year plan & budget with rolling three month forecast).	☐	☐	☐	☐	☐

☐	☐	☐	☐

Team Sizing and Scheduling Work—Development of team sizing models, work schedules & assignments to meet volume I commitment requirements. (Includes development, implementation, assessment and renewal).

| ☐ | ☐ | ☐ | ☐ |

Staffing—Resourcing the team through the selection of new team members, their on boarding, and development plans. Also managing the team member movement to & from the team.

| ☐ | ☐ | ☐ | ☐ |

Processes and Work Clarity—Ensuring team processes & work ownership clarity exists including clarity of responsibility for outputs, activities, tasks & RACI.

| ☐ | ☐ | ☐ | ☐ |

Coaching—Coaching & development of each other on team cultural attributes, norms, member's performance models (critical results & best practices) and over all team leadership skills.

| ☐ | ☐ | ☐ | ☐ |

Team Meetings—Facilitating the team's meetings from developing the agenda, leading the meetings, making sure notes and follow up occur after the meeting while ensuring team participation and ownership of agreements.

| ☐ | ☐ | ☐ | ☐ |

Training and Development—Updating the team on product, policy, process, standards etc. through engaging learning techniques that enhance the teams effectiveness.

| ☐ | ☐ | ☐ | ☐ |

Individual Performance Management—Development and regular review of individual team member's performance and development plans. This includes when necessary dealing with performance problems, establishing performance improvement plans. and making deselection and award recommendations.

| ☐ | ☐ | ☐ | ☐ |

Resource Coordination—Ensures proper coordination with other teams, support groups and partners necessary to complete their work & deliver on the team's commitments.

CAN A TEAM OF LEADERS BREAK THROUGH A HUGE BUREAUCRACY?

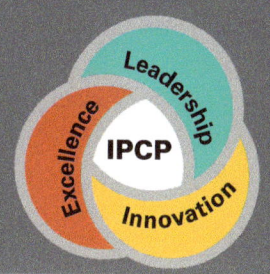

A LARGE GOVERNMENT AGENCY IS DOING POORLY AND MOVING SLOWLY

One of the largest government bureaucracies in the U.S. provides health care and other benefits, including the administration of home mortgages, to military veterans. At the time of this story, this agency had a reputation for being slow and antiquated. In Southern California, not far from Los Angeles, at the agency's regional office, the staff responsible for deciding when veterans are eligible for health care and other benefits was mired in the slow, old ways of doing things.

A NEW LEADER TAKES ON THE PROBLEM

Stew Liff received a call from the agency's western executive asking if he'd lead the Southern California regional office. Stew was an unlikely choice. He'd been trained as a graphic artist and, for most of his career, had been an art teacher in New York City. He didn't have formal business or leadership training. And he'd only recently changed his career direction and joined the government agency as a manager.

Prior to Stew joining the regional office, two top executives had tried to close the office because of its poor performance. Indeed, one of the reasons Stew was chosen for the job is because no other internal leaders would take the job—everyone knew the department was likely to close. So, Stew was basically coming aboard as the new captain of a Titanic.

Stew realized right away that this was going to be a challenging position. Previous leaders had hired employees from the bottom of the labor pool due to the high cost of living in Southern California. Morale was low. And labor-management issues were smoldering. It was no surprise that the regional office had the worst customer satisfaction score in the nation. Other than closing the site, what else could be done?

Source: © Gustavson and Liff (2014). Used with permission. From *A Team of Leaders.*

NOTHING LEFT TO LOSE

Stew quickly learned the office was operating in the same manner as almost every other regional office. It was very hierarchical and comprised of teams that processed claims in an assembly line fashion. After closely examining the situation, Stew decided to try Team of Leaders.

Stew had been your classic "boss in control." He was a leader who made the decisions and told people what to do. So, it was a big move for him to try Team of Leaders. In an ideal world, you'd probably want to implement Team of Leaders with a higher performing organization and a higher level of talent, but Stew didn't have time to make those kinds of change to the organization or staff. Plus, he'd come to feel deep empathy for the employees. He saw that the traditional model frustrated them, stifled innovation and creativity, and led to an incredible amount of waste and rework.

Stew hoped that converting to Team of Leaders would unleash the full potential of the employees, reduce the cynicism of the past 30 years, and bring the focus back onto where it should have been—serving America's heroes.

A ROUGH START

Things didn't start well for Stew and the new approach. There was resistance at all levels. Employees were skeptical and cynical. They feared change and didn't get excited about the opportunity to learn new skill sets. Team leaders felt threatened that they'd lose authority and control.

To make matters worse, two influential employees tried to torpedo the change process. They saw Team of Leaders as being unworkable and made their opinion known, which cast a dark cloud over the process. Moreover, the union representing the employees couldn't understand how union members could adapt to the responsibilities and empowerment that come with Team of Leaders. It didn't help that the team also had to contend with a mountain of claims, a medieval file system, and an immense pressure to perform.

Some wondered if performance might even get worse with the new approach.

BREAKING THROUGH

In Team of Leaders, every team member must understand strategy and execution. Stew was doing his best to make everyone see the big picture, but it wasn't working. That's when he had a brilliant flash—he'd apply his experience as an artist to create visual displays of key metrics and processes. Using this approach let teams see their progress and provided the information they needed to make decisions.

Stew then designed each floor thematically around a war (e.g., the Civil War, World War I, World War II, etc.), and added history displays of each war and each veteran benefit. He also placed centerpieces on each floor (a helicopter, a cannon, a U-2 cockpit, etc.), built private reflection areas (a field hospital, a POW cell, a Vietnam Veterans Memorial, etc.), hung pictures of the faces of veterans from the ceilings, and added patriotic music in the hallways. These displays helped connect the employees to the agency's mission and their customers.

Each team was responsible for designing their work areas to preserve and reinforce their individual uniqueness. This might not seem like a big deal in many organizations, but in a government agency with gray, standard cubes, this was a much-valued touch.

Teams also built "war rooms" to display their overall performance information. Each team had three quarterly improvement goals, and team performance against these goals was posted daily on team monitors. The teams were also encouraged to meet each morning to review performance and come up with ideas for taking the team to a higher level.

THE REGION BECAME A TEAM OF LEADERS

Subtly, Stew's role evolved. He went from being a traditional government bureaucrat to being the conductor of an office symphony. Stew wasn't leading the actual work or solving the problems now. His role was to ensure that all the parts worked together. Team of Leaders had taken hold.

Employees became much more involved and engaged than ever. Many stepped up to provide leadership. And quite a few went on to become national leaders.

Performance improved, with most performance metrics increasing more than 50%. Customer satisfaction also went way up. One important payoff of the new approach was that veterans got help with their mortgage issues, which led to a dramatic decline of property foreclosures. Team members not only went along with the new approach, but they also began to come up with cost saving ideas. Remember, this all began with a low-performing team that was on the verge of being shut down.

Twelve years later, a senior executive says this is the best performing region in the country. Who would have imagined that an art teacher could turn around a completely dysfunctional organization using Team of Leaders and a flair for visualization?

Q&A: WHAT'S THE KEY TO SUCCESS?

Question: If you asked people in the bureaucracy what their job is, what do you think they'd say?

Answer: Team members wouldn't say their job is assisting military veterans. They'd say it's to "always be getting better at assisting veterans." Question: If you asked team members what they think makes their success possible, what would they say? Answer: They'd say it all works because of the trust established between everyone in the agency.

MORE INFORMATION ON STEWART LIFF

Stewart Liff is now an internationally recognized expert on visual management, performance, and team development. He has gone on to become a consultant, speaker, and the author of seven books.

http://stewartliff.com
https://www.linkedin.com/in/stewartliff/
Co-Author, *Team of Leaders*—http://www.ateamofleaders.com

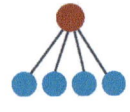 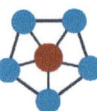 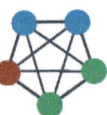 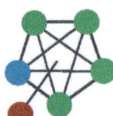 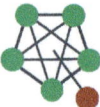

| Stage 1 | Stage 2 | Stage 3 | Stage 4 | Stage 5 |

ABOUT THE TEAM OF LEADERS APPROACH TO TEAM LEADERSHIP

Becoming a Team of Leaders is a powerful but different approach to leading teams. Many of us learned that high-performing teams require strong, decisive, take-charge leadership. In this traditional model, the team leader plans, organizes, and distributes work—he or she is the "center" of all teamwork. With Team of Leaders, all team members share the team's leadership responsibilities. Topics and decisions that the team leader once handled on his or her own are now released to team members when they're prepared and ready to take them on. This approach allows the team leader to "scale up" and spend more time making strategic and cross-functional contributions.

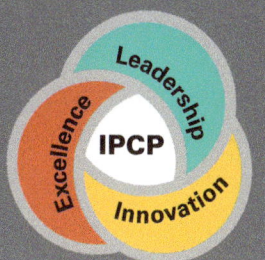

UNITED STATES OF AMERICA (THE)

GII 2019 rank

3

Output rank	Input rank	Income	Region	Population (mn)	GDP, PPP$	GDP per capita, PPP$	GII 2018 rank
6	3	High	NAC	326.8	20,513.0	62,605.6	6

		Score/Value	Rank	
	INSTITUTIONS	**89.7**	**11**	
1.1	**Political environment**	**84.2**	**16**	
1.1.1	Political and operational stability*	84.2	25	
1.1.2	Government effectiveness*	84.2	14	
1.2	**Regulatory environment**	**93.9**	**9**	
1.2.1	Regulatory quality*	85.6	15	
1.2.2	Rule of law*	89.9	15	
1.2.3	Cost of redundancy dismissal, salary weeks	8.0	1	●
1.3	**Business environment**	**91.1**	**2**	● ◆
1.3.1	Ease of starting a business*	91.2	47	
1.3.2	Ease of resolving insolvency*	90.9	3	● ◆

		Score/Value	Rank	
	HUMAN CAPITAL & RESEARCH	**55.7**	**12**	
2.1	**Education**	**54.5**	**45**	
2.1.1	Expenditure on education, % GDP	5.0	50	
2.1.2	Government funding/pupil, secondary, % GDP/cap.	22.5	39	
2.1.3	School life expectancy, years	16.3	29	
2.1.4	PISA scales in reading, maths, & science	487.6	29	◇
2.1.5	Pupil-teacher ratio, secondary	14.7	67	○ ◇
2.2	**Tertiary education**	**34.6**	**53**	
2.2.1	Tertiary enrolment, % gross	88.8	8	
2.2.2	Graduates in science & engineering, %	17.9	73	○
2.2.3	Tertiary inbound mobility, %	5.0	40	
2.3	**Research & development (R&D)**	**77.9**	**3**	● ◆
2.3.1	Researchers, FTE/mn pop.	4,256.3	23	
2.3.2	Gross expenditure on R&D, % GDP	2.8	9	
2.3.3	Global R&D companies, avg. exp. top 3, mn US$	100.0	1	● ◆
2.3.4	QS university ranking, average score top 3*	99.0	1	● ◆

		Score/Value	Rank	
	INFRASTRUCTURE	**59.2**	**23**	
3.1	**Information & communication technologies(ICTs)**	**89.7**	**8**	
3.1.1	ICT access*	84.8	14	
3.1.2	ICT use*	77.2	21	
3.1.3	Government's online service*	98.6	2	●
3.1.4	E-participation*	98.3	5	
3.2	**General infrastructure**	**49.4**	**19**	
3.2.1	Electricity output, kWh/mn pop.	13,000.9	9	
3.2.2	Logistics performance*	85.2	14	
3.2.3	Gross capital formation, % GDP	21.1	87	○
3.3	**Ecological sustainability**	**38.4**	**64**	◇
3.3.1	GDP/unit of energy use	8.1	74	○
3.3.2	Environmental performance*	71.2	26	
3.3.3	ISO 14001 environmental certificates/bn PPP$ GDP	0.3	106	○ ◇

		Score/Value	Rank	
	MARKET SOPHISTICATION	**87.0**	**1**	● ◆
4.1	**Credit**	**94.6**	**1**	● ◆
4.1.1	Ease of getting credit*	95.0	3	● ◆
4.1.2	Domestic credit to private sector, % GDP	192.2	3	● ◆
4.1.3	Microfinance gross loans, % GDP	n/a	n/a	
4.2	**Investment**	**73.7**	**7**	◆
4.2.1	Ease of protecting minority investors*	64.7	47	
4.2.2	Market capitalization, % GDP	150.3	5	
4.2.3	Venture capital deals/bn PPP$ GDP	0.4	1	● ◆
4.3	**Trade, competition, & market scale**	**92.7**	**1**	● ◆
4.3.1	Applied tariff rate, weighted avg., %	1.7	18	
4.3.2	Intensity of local competition†	84.3	3	● ◆
4.3.3	Domestic market scale, bn PPP$	20,513.0	2	● ◆

		Score/Value	Rank	
	BUSINESS SOPHISTICATION	**62.7**	**7**	
5.1	**Knowledge workers**	**76.4**	**4**	◆
5.1.1	Knowledge-intensive employment, %	47.3	11	
5.1.2	Firms offering formal training, % firms	n/a	n/a	
5.1.3	GERD performed by business, % GDP	2.0	8	
5.1.4	GERD financed by business, %	63.6	9	
5.1.5	Females employed w/advanced degrees, %	26.3	6	◆
5.2	**Innovation linkages**	**54.3**	**9**	
5.2.1	University/industry research collaboration†	80.9	1	● ◆
5.2.2	State of cluster development†	79.5	1	● ◆
5.2.3	GERD financed by abroad, %	6.2	58	○
5.2.4	JV-strategic alliance deals/bn PPP$ GDP	0.1	9	
5.2.5	Patent families 2+ offices/bn PPP$ GDP	3.3	15	
5.3	**Knowledge absorption**	**57.3**	**7**	
5.3.1	Intellectual property payments, % total trade	1.8	15	
5.3.2	High-tech imports, % total trade	17.2	9	◆
5.3.3	ICT services imports, % total trade	1.5	40	
5.3.4	FDI net inflows, % GDP	2.4	72	○
5.3.5	Research talent, % in business enterprise	71.0	5	◆

		Score/Value	Rank	
	KNOWLEDGE & TECHNOLOGY OUTPUTS	**59.7**	**4**	◆
6.1	**Knowledge creation**	**72.3**	**3**	● ◆
6.1.1	Patents by origin/bn PPP$ GDP	15.1	6	◆
6.1.2	PCT patents by origin/bn PPP$ GDP	2.7	12	
6.1.3	Utility models by origin/bn PPP$ GDP	n/a	n/a	
6.1.4	Scientific & technical articles/bn PPP$ GDP	10.5	44	◇
6.1.5	Citable documents H-index	100.0	1	● ◆
6.2	**Knowledge impact**	**60.4**	**2**	● ◆
6.2.1	Growth rate of PPP$ GDP/worker, %	0.9	64	○
6.2.2	New businesses/th pop. 15-64	n/a	n/a	
6.2.3	Computer software spending, % GDP	1.1	1	● ◆
6.2.4	ISO 9001 quality certificates/bn PPP$ GDP	1.5	99	○ ◇
6.2.5	High- & medium-high-tech manufactures, %	0.5	10	
6.3	**Knowledge diffusion**	**46.5**	**15**	
6.3.1	Intellectual property receipts, % total trade	5.0	1	● ◆
6.3.2	High-tech net exports, % total trade	5.8	27	
6.3.3	ICT services exports, % total trade	1.6	65	
6.3.4	FDI net outflows, % GDP	1.8	33	

		Score/Value	Rank	
	CREATIVE OUTPUTS	**45.5**	**15**	
7.1	**Intangible assets**	**50.3**	**32**	
7.1.1	Trademarks by origin/bn PPP$ GDP	22.0	85	○ ◇
7.1.2	Industrial designs by origin/bn PPP$ GDP	1.2	61	
7.1.3	ICTs & business model creation†	81.0	6	
7.1.4	ICTs & organizational model creation†	83.7	1	● ◆
7.2	**Creative goods & services**	**43.8**	**5**	◆
7.2.1	Cultural & creative services exports, % total trade	2.5	5	◆
7.2.2	National feature films/mn pop. 15-69	2.9	58	
7.2.3	Entertainment & Media market/th pop. 15-69	100.0	1	● ◆
7.2.4	Printing & other media, % manufacturing	1.5	31	
7.2.5	Creative goods exports, % total trade	3.3	17	
7.3	**Online creativity**	**37.5**	**19**	
7.3.1	Generic top-level domains (TLDs)/th pop. 15-69	100.0	1	● ◆
7.3.2	Country-code TLDs/th pop. 15-69	2.4	62	◇
7.3.3	Wikipedia edits/mn pop. 15-69	26.1	42	◇
7.3.4	Mobile app creation/bn PPP$ GDP	30.1	17	

NOTES: ● indicates a strength; ○ a weakness; ◆ a strength relative to the other top 25-ranked GII economies; ◇ a weakness relative to the other top 25-ranked GII economies; * an index; † a survey question. ⊕ indicates that the economy's data are older than the base year; see Appendix II for details, including the year of the data, at http://globalinnovationindex.org. Square brackets [ ] indicate that the data minimum coverage (DMC) requirements were not met at the sub-pillar or pillar level.

INNOVATOR AND
COGNITIVE BIAS WORKSHEETS

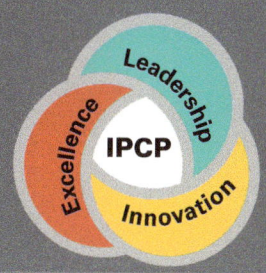

DISRUPTORS

> **"** …Innovators rely on their 'courage to innovate' – an active bias against the status quo and an unflinching willingness to take smart risks – to transform ideas into powerful impact. **"**
>
> Jeff Dyer and Hal Gregersen (2012)
> American Management Association.

Innovator Worksheet:
Mastering the Five Skills of Disruptive Innovators

Associating–The ability to connect seemingly unrelated questions, problems or ideas from different fields, 'connecting the dots to Ding the Universe'

Questioning–Constantly ask questions that challenge common wisdom coupled with a desire to change the world, Asks "Why?", "Why not?" and "What if?"

Observing–Produce uncommon ideas by scrutinizing common phenomena, particularly the behavior of potential customers – conduct 'anthropological digging'

Experimenting–Actively try out new ideas by creating prototypes and launching pilots-they make experimentation central to what they do, encouraging the pursuit of 'blind alleys'

Networking–Finding and testing new ideas through a network of diverse people to gain a radically different perspective, nurturing opportunities to experience 'AHA! Moments'

Cognitive Bias Worksheet:

A partial check-list to help you think about common bias influences.

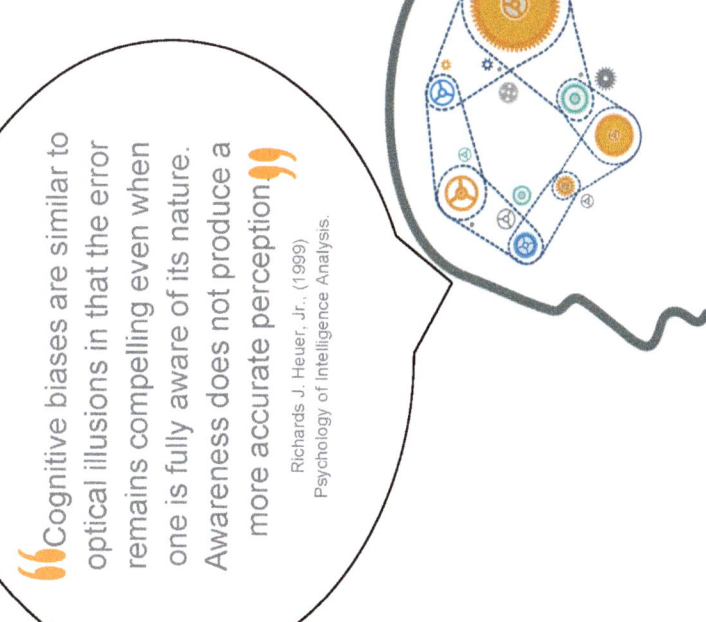

❝Cognitive biases are similar to optical illusions in that the error remains compelling even when one is fully aware of its nature. Awareness does not produce a more accurate perception❞

Richards J. Heuer, Jr., (1999)
Psychology of Intelligence Analysis.

☐ Anchoring Bias: A tendency to compare and contrast only a limited set of items – we fixate on a value or number that gets compared to everything else

☐ Belief Bias: A biasing effect of personal knowledge on judgments

☐ Bias Blind Spot: People think biases are more prevalent in others

☐ Confirmation Bias: A tendency to seek confirmation from one's convictions, fueling our preconceived views while ignoring or dismissing opinions that threaten our world view

☐ Gamblers Fallacy: We tend to put a lot of weight on previous events which distorts reality about probabilities

☐ Groupthink: Striving for consensus at the cost of a realistic appraisal of alternative actions

☐ Negativity Bias: Paying attention to bad news because we perceive it to be more important or credible

☐ Overconfidence Bias: Overestimating our skill levels relative to others, leading us to overestimate our ability to affect future outcomes– chance is neglected

☐ Projection Bias: Assuming most people think like us and agree with us–overestimation of how 'typical' we are

☐ Status Quo Bias: Preference for the status quo in the absence of pressure to change it, "If it ain't broke don't fix it" thinking

BIG DATA
TEAM LEVEL COMPETENCY

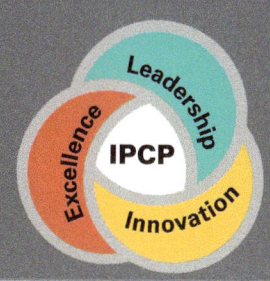

Big Data Team Level Competency

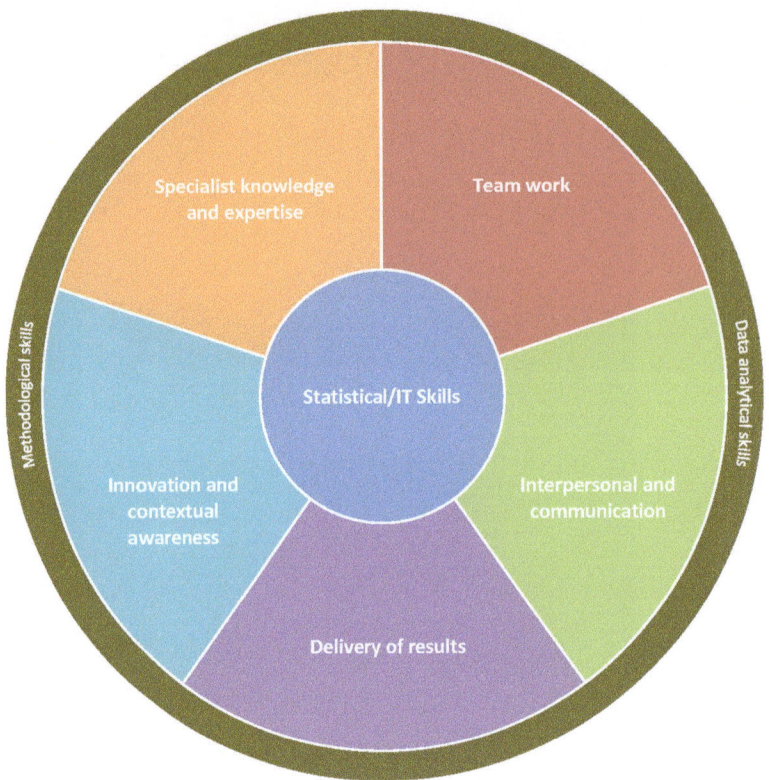

Team work	Ability to work collaboratively with others, developing and maintaining good working relationships and sharing information and knowledge
Interpersonal and communication	The ability to communicate with others in a fluent, logical, clear and convincing manner together with an ability to engage effectively with a wide range of stakeholders
Delivery of results	Ability to deliver outcomes on time and to a high standard and ensure that goals are achieved
Innovation and contextual awareness	Ability to observe environmental factors and exploit them for the work environment together with the ability to develop new ideas, concepts and solutions outside of established patterns
Specialist knowledge and expertise	Possess appropriate specialist knowledge and expertise to work effectively as part of the Big Data team
Statistical/IT skills	Possess detailed knowledge and understanding of statistical methodology and concepts, ability to extract key messages or underlying trends within data and possess the IT skills relevant to statistical production and analysis
Data Analytical/ Visualisation skills	Ability to work with structured and unstructured data and combine data processing techniques to achieve outcomes, possess knowledge and understanding of data visualization techniques relevant to big data

Big Data Team Level Competencies – *Performance indicators*

Team work	
	Shows respect for colleagues and co-workers
	Supports colleagues and takes views of others on board
	Is adaptive and works to achieve common goals
	Is able to work with a group of people in a constructive way and can motivate others
	Weighs information from all sources including team before making decisions

Interpersonal and communication	
	Presents information clearly, concisely and confidently when speaking and in writing
	Projects conviction, gaining buy in by outlining relevant information and selling the benefits
	Develops and maintains networks of contacts to facilitate problem solving or information sharing
	Treats others with diplomacy, tact courtesy and respect, even in challenging circumstances
	Takes into account different views/perspectives and forms opinion on the basis of information and discussions

Delivery of results	
	Maintains a strong focus on the ultimate goal and works to achieve this
	Sets measurable, achievable and clear objectives on own work
	Uses resources effectively, challenging processes to improve efficiencies
	Looks critically at issues to see how things could be done better
	Applies appropriate systems/controls to deliver efficient and high value results

Innovation and contextual awareness	
	Awareness of environmental factors that could affect current policy
	Has the skill to translate external developments into statistical indicators
	Integrates diverse strands of information, identifying inter-relationships and linkages
	Is resourceful and creative, generating original approaches when solving problems and making decisions
	Comes up with innovative ideas and thinks unconventionally about questions or problems
	Challenges the established wisdom and adopts an open minded approach coming up with new solutions

Specialist knowledge and expertise	
	Clearly understands the role, objectives and targets and how they fit into the work of the team
	Develops the expertise necessary to carry out the role to a high standard and shares this with others
	Has significant expertise in own field that is recognised and utilised by colleagues
	Is proactive in keeping up to date on issues and key developments that may impact on own area and office generally
	Ability to work with structured, unstructured and semi-structured data and ability to categorise data
	Ability to process data in batch and streaming modes
	Understanding of data base models associated with big data such as relational document, big value, NewSQL etc.
	Understanding of security and privacy issues associated with big data

Statistical/IT skills	
	Is able to use core statistical skills for data analysis such as: quantitative and qualitative analysis, weighting, inference, validity and modeling
	Can use programming/scripting languages associated with statistical computing environments such as R, SAS, SPSS or equivalent
	Can combine various data processing techniques to achieve given analytical task
	Good knowledge of data science and data science methods
	Shows evidence of keeping up to date with new trends in data techniques and technologies
	Ability to process and generate large data sets using an appropriate programming model such as MapReduce
	Ability to use stream process technologies such as Apache Storm, MapR etc.
	Ability to use batch process technologies such as Hadoop
	Ability to use open source cluster computing systems such as Spark
	Ability to use tools associated with machine learning algorithms such as regression, classification, cluster and dimensionality reduction

Data Analytical/ Visualisation skills	
	Strong ability to work with appropriate coding/scripting languages
	Ability to develop software for more advanced data processing tasks
	Can use high performance computing platforms in an efficient way
	Can operate on structured and unstructured data with a wide range of tools
	Ability to analyse complex data and identify what is relevant
	Can combine various data processing techniques to achieve a given analytical task
	Can assimilate information from a range of sources and organise complex information to make it accessible
	Understanding of machine learning algorithms such as supervised and unsupervised learning, semi-supervised classification and reinforced learning
	Ability to apply data mining techniques to unstructured data sets such as time-series data, streaming data, sequence data, graph data, spatial data and multimedia data
	Understanding of data visualisation techniques under the broad headings of spatial layout visualisation, abstract/summary visualisation and real time interactive visualisation

NURSING INFORMATION LITERACY AND CRITICAL THINKING SELF-ASSESSMENT

INSTRUCTIONS

For each Performance indicator included in the ACRL Nursing Information Literacy Competencies Standard 3 you see specific outcome Knowledge, Skills, and Attitudes (KSA's) associated with a performance indicator. Rate yourself on how you can apply your critical thinking skills to achieve each KSA outcome.

Step 1: Print out the Assessment (legal size paper required).

Step 2: Reflect on the Performance Outcomes for each indicator. For each indicator self-assess your critical thinking abilities to achieve those outcomes. A Performance Indicator often has more than one Critical Thinking KSA to consider. Circle the description that best represents your competencies for each Critical Thinking KSA category denoted in orange.

Step 3: Once you complete the self-assessment take 15 minutes and reflect on your responses. Note items you rated high (4) and low (1 or 2). Consider: Based on your responses, what support would you need to feel comfortable participating in an interdisciplinary big data analytics team that was responsible to use big data to make patient care recommendations?

Step 4: Save your results and be prepared to share your thoughts during the live discussion.

Critical Thinking Standards and Measures

Used with permission from the Foundation for Critical Thinking's rubrics for assessing student reasoning abilities (2013). Retrieved from http://www.criticalthinking.org.

1.   Thinking is unskilled and insufficient, marked by imprecision, lack of clarity, superficiality, illogicality, and inaccuracy, and unfairness

2.   Thinking is inconsistent, ineffective; shows a lack of consistent competence: is often unclear, imprecise, inaccurate, and superficial

3.   Thinking is competent, effective, accurate and clear, but lacks the exemplary depth, precision, and insight of a 4

4.   Thinking is exemplary, skilled, marked by excellence in clarity, accuracy, precision, relevance, depth, breadth, logicality, and fairness

Nursing Information Literacy Standards

Performance indicators from ACRL Information Literacy Competency Standards for Nursing used with permission of the Association of College and Research Libraries(ACRL), a division of the American Library Association. These standards are integrated into the TIGER standards for Nursing Informatics.

ACRL Nursing Information Literacy Competency Standards for Nursing—Standard 3

The information literate nurse critically evaluates the procured information and its sources, and as a result, decides whether or not to modify the initial query and/or seek additional sources and whether to develop a new research process.

Performance Indicators	4 - Exemplary	3 - Satisfactory	2 - Below Satisfactory	1 - Unsatisfactory
The information literate nurse:	If applicable, consistently does all or almost all of the following	If applicable, consistently does most or many of the following	If applicable, consistently does most or many of the following	If applicable, consistently does all or almost all of the following
1. Summarizes the main ideas to be extracted from the information gathered.		**PURPOSE**		
Outcomes include:	Demonstrates a clear understanding of the assignment's [or data results] purpose	Demonstrates an understanding of the assignment's [or data results] purpose	Is not completely clear about the purpose of the assignment [or data results]	Does not clearly understand the purpose of the assignment [or data results]
		KEY QUESTION, PROBLEM, OR ISSUE		
a. Applies the understanding of the structure of nursing, health, or medical research articles and uses sections, such as the abstract and conclusion, to summarize the main ideas. b. Selects main ideas from the text. c. Identifies the elements of the question addressed, and/or restates the main ideas of the information source to address the question. d. Identifies verbatim material that can then be appropriately quoted.	--Clearly defines the issue or problem; accurately identifies the core issues --Appreciates depth and breadth of problem --Demonstrates fair-mindedness toward problem	--Defines the issue; identifies the core issues, but may not fully explore their depth and breadth --Demonstrates fair-mindedness	--Defines the issue, but poorly (superficially, narrowly); may overlook some core issues --Has trouble maintaining a fair-minded approach toward the problem	--Fails to clearly define the issue or problem; does not recognize the core issues --Fails to maintain a fair-minded approach toward the problem

| Performance Indicators

The information literate nurse: | 4 - Exemplary

If applicable, consistently does all or almost all of the following | 3 - Satisfactory

If applicable, consistently does most or many of the following | 2- Below Satisfactory

If applicable, consistently does most or many of the following | 1 - Unsatisfactory

If applicable, consistently does all or almost all of the following |
|---|---|---|---|---|
| **2. Selects information by articulating and applying criteria for evaluating both the information and its sources.** | | POINT OF VIEW | | |
| Outcomes include:

a. Distinguishes among facts, points of view, and opinion. | --Identifies and evaluates relevant significant points of view | --Identifies and evaluates relevant points of view | --May identify other points of view but struggles with maintaining fairmindedness; may focus on irrelevant or insignificant points of view | --Ignores or superficially evaluates alternate points of view |
b. Differentiates clinical opinion from research and evidence summaries.	--Is empathetic, fair in examining all relevant points of view	--Is fair in examining those views		--Cannot separate own vested interests and feelings when evaluating other points of view
c. Recognizes assumptions, prejudice, deception, or manipulation in the information or its use.		INFORMATION		
d. Considers resources from a variety of disciplines beyond nursing, including education and teaching, psychology, business, leadership and management, public health, health care administration, demographics, and social sciences.	--Gathers sufficient, credible, relevant information: observations, statements, logic, data, facts, questions, graphs, themes, assertions, descriptions, etc.	--Gathers sufficient, credible, and relevant information	--Gathers some credible information, but not enough; some information may be irrelevant	--Relies on insufficient, irrelevant, or unreliable information
e. Examines and compares information and evidence from various sources in order to evaluate reliability, validity, accuracy, authority, currency, and point of view or bias.	--Includes information that opposes as well as supports the argued position	--Includes some information from opposing views	--Omits significant information, including some strong counter-arguments	--Fails to identify or hastily dismisses strong, relevant counter-arguments
f. Recognizes the cultural, historical, physical, political, social, or other context within which the information was created, and understands the impact of context on interpreting the information.	--Distinguishes between information and inferences drawn from that information	--Distinguishes between information and inferences drawn from it	--Sometimes confuses information and the inferences drawn from it	--Confuses information and inferences drawn from that information
g. Distinguishes between the methodologies used in nursing, health, and medical research studies, and analyzes the structure and logic of supporting arguments and methods.				
h. Identifies gaps in the literature as research opportunities.				

Performance Indicators	4 - Exemplary	3 - Satisfactory	2 - Below Satisfactory	1 - Unsatisfactory
The information literate nurse:	If applicable, consistently does all or almost all of the following	If applicable, consistently does most or many of the following	If applicable, consistently does most or many of the following	If applicable, consistently does all or almost all of the following
3. Synthesizes main ideas to construct new concepts.			CONCEPTS	
Outcomes include:				
a. Synthesizes divergent information to answer a research question and generalizes relative research to a related question.	--Identifies and accurately explains/uses the relevant key concepts	--Identifies and accurately explains and uses the key concepts, but not with the depth and precision of a "4"	--Identifies some (not all) key concepts, but use of concepts is superficial and inaccurate at times	--Misunderstands key concepts or ignores relevant key concepts altogether
b. Recognizes interrelationships among concepts and combines them into potentially useful primary statements and/or summary of findings with supporting evidence.			INFORMATION	
c. Extends initial synthesis, when possible, at a higher level of abstraction to construct new hypotheses that may require additional information.	--Gathers sufficient, credible, relevant information: observations, statements, logic, data, facts, questions, graphs, themes, assertions, descriptions, etc.	--Gathers sufficient, credible, and relevant information	--Gathers some credible information, but not enough; some information may be irrelevant	--Relies on insufficient, irrelevant, or unreliable information
d. Utilizes computer and other technologies (e.g. spreadsheets, databases, multimedia, simulators, and audio or visual equipment) for studying the interaction of ideas and other phenomena.				
e. Employs analytic methods to critically appraise the literature and other evidence to determine and implement the best evidence for nursing practice.	--Includes information that opposes as well as supports the argued position	--Includes some information from opposing views	--Omits significant information, including some strong counter-arguments	--Fails to identify or hastily dismisses strong, relevant counter-arguments
f. Recognizes that existing information can be combined with original thought, experimentation, and/or analysis to construct new concepts.	--Distinguishes between information and inferences drawn from that information	--Distinguishes between information and inferences drawn from it	--Sometimes confuses information and the inferences drawn from it	--Confuses information and inferences drawn from that information
g. Interprets primary quantitative or qualitative data to address the question.				

Performance Indicators	4 - Exemplary	3 - Satisfactory	2 - Below Satisfactory	1 - Unsatisfactory
The information literate nurse:	If applicable, consistently does all or almost all of the following	If applicable, consistently does most or many of the following	If applicable, consistently does most or many of the following	If applicable, consistently does all or almost all of the following
4. Compares new knowledge with prior knowledge to determine the value added, contradictions, or other unique characteristics of the information.		ASSUMPTIONS		
Outcomes include:	--Accurately identifies assumptions (things taken for granted)	--Identifies assumptions	--Fails to identify assumptions, or fails to explain them, or the assumptions identified are irrelevant, not clearly stated, and/or invalid	--Fails to identify assumptions
a. Values the need for continuous improvement based on new knowledge.	--Makes assumptions that are consistent, reasonable, valid	--Makes valid assumptions		--Makes invalid assumptions
b. Discriminates between valid and invalid reasons for modifying evidence-based practice.				
c. Uses consciously selected criteria to determine whether the information contradicts or verifies information used from other sources.		INFORMATION		
	--Gathers sufficient, credible, relevant information: observations, statements, logic, data, facts, questions, graphs, themes, assertions, descriptions, etc.	--Gathers sufficient, credible, and relevant information	--Gathers some credible information, but not enough; some information may be irrelevant	--Relies on insufficient, irrelevant, or unreliable information
d. Draws conclusions based upon information gathered.				
e. Tests theories with discipline-appropriate techniques (e.g., simulators, experiments).	--Includes information that opposes as well as supports the argued position	--Includes some information from opposing views	--Omits significant information, including some strong counter-arguments	--Fails to identify or hastily dismisses strong, relevant counter-arguments
f. Determines probable accuracy by questioning the source of the information, limitations of the information gathering tools or strategies, and the reasonableness of the conclusions.	--Distinguishes between information and inferences drawn from that information	--Distinguishes between information and inferences drawn from it	--Sometimes confuses information and the inferences drawn from it	--Confuses information and inferences drawn from that information
g. Integrates new information with previous information or knowledge.		INTERPRETATIONS, INFERENCES		
h. Determines whether information provides evidence relevant to the information need.	--Follows where evidence and reason lead in order to obtain defensible, thoughtful, logical conclusions or solutions	--Follows where evidence and reason lead to obtain justifiable, logical conclusions	--Does follow some evidence to conclusions, but inferences are more often than not unclear, illogical, inconsistent, and/or superficial	--Uses superficial, simplistic, or irrelevant reasons and unjustifiable claims
i. Includes information that is pertinent even when it contradicts the individual's value system, being careful to maintain a neutral position.	--Makes deep rather than superficial inferences	--Makes valid inferences, but not with the same depth and as a "4"		--Makes illogical, inconsistent inferences
	--Makes inferences that are consistent with one another			--Exhibits closed-mindedness or hostility to reason; regardless of the evidence, maintains or defends views based on self-interest

Performance Indicators	4 - Exemplary	3 - Satisfactory	2 - Below Satisfactory	1 - Unsatisfactory
The information literate nurse:	If applicable, consistently does all or almost all of the following	If applicable, consistently does most or many of the following	If applicable, consistently does most or many of the following	If applicable, consistently does all or almost all of the following
5. Validates understanding and interpretation of the information through discourse with other individuals, subject-area experts, and/or practitioners.	POINT OF VIEW			
Outcomes include:				
a. Participates in classroom and virtual/electronic discussions for validating understanding and interpreting the information.	--Identifies and evaluates relevant significant points of view	--Identifies and evaluates relevant points of view	--May identify other points of view but struggles with maintaining fairmindedness; may focus on irrelevant or insignificant points of view	--Ignores or superficially evaluates alternate points of view
b. Works effectively in small groups or teams.	--Is empathetic, fair in examining all relevant points of view	--Is fair in examining those views		--Cannot separate own vested interests and feelings when evaluating other points of view
c. Seeks expert opinion through a variety of mechanisms (e.g., interviews, electronic communication).	IMPLICATIONS, CONSEQUENCES			
	--Identifies the most significant implications and consequences of the reasoning (whether positive and/or negative)	--Identifies significant implications and consequences and distinguishes probable from improbable implications, but not with the same insight and precision as a "4"	--Has trouble identifying significant implications and consequences; identifies improbable implications	--Ignores significant implications and consequences of reasoning
d. Utilizes, and/or contributes to, and shares evidence of best practices with, interprofessional teams.	--Distinguishes probable from improbable implications			
e. Initiates and facilitates professional discourse and discussions as a team member, mentor, practitioner, preceptor, and/or educator.				

Your Comments/Notes:

Performance Indicators The information literate nurse:	4 - Exemplary If applicable, consistently does all or almost all of the following	3 - Satisfactory If applicable, consistently does most or many of the following	2- Below Satisfactory If applicable, consistently does most or many of the following	1 - Unsatisfactory If applicable, consistently does all or almost all of the following
6. Determines whether the initial query should be revised.				
Outcomes include:		CONCEPTS		
	--Identifies and accurately explains/uses the relevant key concepts	--Identifies and accurately explains and uses the key concepts, but not with the depth and precision of a "4"	--Identifies some (not all) key concepts, but use of concepts is superficial and inaccurate at times	--Misunderstands key concepts or ignores relevant key concepts altogether
a. Participates in peer review of search [and data] strategies with information professionals, students, nurses, and/or faculty. b. Draws conclusions based on a combination of personal training and research. c. Determines if original information need has been satisfied or if additional information is needed. d. Reviews search [and data] strategy and incorporates additional concepts as necessary. e. Reviews information retrieval [and data] sources used and expands to include others as needed.		IMPLICATIONS, CONSEQUENCES		
	--Identifies the most significant implications and consequences of the reasoning (whether positive and/or negative) --Distinguishes probable from improbable implications --Demonstrates fair-mindedness toward problem	--Identifies significant implications and consequences and distinguishes probable from improbable implications, but not with the same insight and precision as a "4"	--Has trouble identifying significant implications and consequences; identifies improbable implications	--Ignores significant implications and consequences of reasoning

Performance Indicators	4 - Exemplary	3 - Satisfactory	2 - Below Satisfactory	1 - Unsatisfactory
The information literate nurse:	If applicable, consistently does all or almost all of the following	If applicable, consistently does most or many of the following	If applicable, consistently does most or many of the following	If applicable, consistently does all or almost all of the following
7. Evaluates the procured information and the entire process.	KEY QUESTION, PROBLEM, OR ISSUE			
Outcomes include: a. Reviews and assesses the procured information and determines possible improvements in the information seeking process. b. Applies the improvements to subsequent projects.	--Clearly defines the issue or problem; accurately identifies the core issues --Appreciates depth and breadth of problem --Demonstrates fair-mindedness toward problem	--Defines the issue; identifies the core issues, but may not fully explore their depth and breadth --Demonstrates fair-mindedness	--Defines the issue, but poorly (superficially, narrowly); may overlook some core issues --Has trouble maintaining a fair-minded approach toward the problem	--Fails to clearly define the issue or problem; does not recognize the core issues --Fails to maintain a fair-minded approach toward the problem

Your Comments/Notes: